17 95

Enjoy the book!

Shirley
Bellinger

D1499582

INNER EATING

INNER EATING

SHIRLEY BILLIGMEIER

A Division of Thomas Nelson Publishers
Nashville

Published in Nashville, Tennessee, by Oliver-Nelson Books, a division of Thomas Nelson, Inc., Publishers, and distributed in Canada by Lawson Falle, Ltd., Cambridge, Ontario.

Basic food groups chart from FIT-OR-FAT TARGET DIET by Covert Bailey. Copyright © 1984 by Covert Bailey. Reprinted by permission of Houghton Mifflin Co.

CATHY Cartoons in chapters 4 and 16 are COPYRIGHT 1989 UNIVERSAL PRESS SYNDICATE. Reprinted with permission. All rights reserved.

Cartoon in chapter 16 copyright 1977 and reprinted by permission of Jules Feiffer.

Unless otherwise noted, the Bible version used in this publication is THE NEW KING JAMES VERSION. Copyright © 1979, 1980, 1982, Thomas Nelson, Inc., Publishers.

Library of Congress Cataloging-in-Publication Data

Billigmeier, Shirley, 1950–
      Inner eating / Shirley Billigmeier.
          p.   cm.
      Includes bibliographical references.
      ISBN 0-8407-9113-5
      1. Reducing.   2. Food habits.   3. Appetite disorders.   I. Title.
RM222.2.B55   1991
613.2′5—dc20   90–49616
                                                                                             CIP

Printed in the United States of America.
ISBN 0-8407-9113-5

                                    1 2 3 4 5 6 — 96 95 94 93 92 91

To my husband,
Jon,
who lived the process
before I created it.

To my children,
Katie and Steve,
who are thrilled the book
is finished!

Contents

Foreword

I rarely advise patients seeking advice on weight control to go on a diet. The reason is simple. A "diet" is something people do until it works, until it fails, or until they get tired of it. They then return to doing what it was that made it necessary for them to go on a diet in the first place.

People become overweight because they have the genetic ability to readily turn extra calories into fat (not everyone does) and they eat sufficient amounts of high fat food and get too little physical activity. The United States, unfortunately, provides an excellent environment for the latter requirements.

Despite too little exercise and readily available food, however, the majority of people do not consistently eat more than they burn. Thus, they maintain their weight at a healthy level. Even for those individuals who do gain excess weight it is now becoming clear that not all weight gain is equally unhealthy, nor is weight likely to be gained for the same reasons.

In *Inner Eating,* Shirley Billigmeier addresses issues of appropriate eating that are quite relevant for certain groups of people. She has learned from the experiences of herself, her friends, and her clients what doesn't work (diets) and has made important insights into what may help the chronically frustrated dieter. She points out that eating should serve only to nourish the body and provide enjoyment to the eater. A number of people have lost sight of one or both of these points.

She emphasizes that this group of people must learn to admit to and define each act of eating and listen to their bodies. Obviously, there are many steps to be taken and issues to be addressed to accomplish these goals. Ms. Billigmeier has carefully outlined her approach for helping people focus on learning how to eat to be satisfied. By using examples from some of her clients, she brings up and addresses many issues that frustrate people's ability to take control of their eating habits.

If you are the type of chronic, frustrated dieter the author is addressing (see the test on page 21) it's likely you will learn something about yourself by reading this book. I hope, as does Ms. Billigmeier, that this process of learning will enable you to be satisfied with your body.

MICHAEL D. JENSEN, M.D.
Associate Professor of Medicine
The Mayo Clinic

Preface

Our core issue in this book and for anyone with eating problems is the *act of eating*. That is the focus, finally, of all eating problems: what you put in your mouth, chew, and swallow. The other issues (emotions, taste, etc.) influence your act of eating, but they have no calories in themselves. Therefore, my aim is to help you separate your act of eating from all other peripheral issues and own that act and take charge of it.

First, you'll learn to recognize the act of eating. Doesn't that sound silly? But it's true. We lose the ability to recognize eating, whether we put food in our mouths because we're actually hungry or because we've been in an emotionally disturbing situation.

Second, you'll realize that you have a choice. That is probably the overriding feature of Inner Eating next to identifying the act of eating. The choice to begin, to continue, and to change anything you wish regarding your eating is within your power. It's internal and belongs to no one else. Ownership is your inherent right, and the motor that drives Inner Eating.

Third, you'll learn to recognize some of your emotional issues. I don't pretend to be able to fix them, but your awareness of their existence is a major step because it empowers you to take charge of an area that, until now, was a vast unknown for you. Then you can work through those issues.

Fourth, after discovering some of your issues, you'll want to know how to pass this gift of freedom on to your family. I'll show you some ways to do that. Then we'll talk about the other end of the eating disorder scale, self-starvation and bingeing, and how it relates to the act of eating.

Finally, you'll gain knowledge about physical fitness and body image and how it all ties together to help you see yourself as a whole person. Even with physical limitations, you can tone your body.

The result of this process is to allow you to value and honor yourself as a unique person with a particular set of likes and dislikes that—if it is valid—you can change or modify as you choose.

That freedom makes some people afraid, and they seek external controls for the comfort and predictability they offer. With Inner Eating you will learn that it's not a matter of will and other-control but of cherishing the divine gift of life that is your body. Your beautiful body is managed ultimately by your brain. And, again, ultimately it's your responsibility, and no other person's. External control is different from internal choice in that inner choice gives strength and wisdom, self-revelation and self-respect, clarity and freedom. As you give yourself those gifts, you will learn who you are, and *there is no greater gift that you can give yourself, than the gift of yourself.* As you honor that gift, you honor the Giver.

I believe that God is the giver of all life, and with life comes the body signals and instincts also, His special gifts to us, that we are responsible for listening to. No external control can do that. If we fight against those instincts by ignoring them or by refusing to listen to their messages to us, we do a disservice to our bodies and to our own well-being. In effect we begin to disfigure and mar His creation (our bodies), often at terrible cost to us and to others. That willfulness honors neither the gift nor the Giver. That sentiment, on which rests the whole of Inner Eating, is celebrated through this text with Notes to Myself. My greatest joy has been to give the discoveries of Inner Eating to my clients. It is my gift to you.

SHIRLEY BILLIGMEIER

Acknowledgments

This work represents a ten-year journey. Without the help of a fine team of professionals, I would not have been able to share my gift.

These people and many more were all part of the creative force of this manuscript:

Victor Oliver, who saw the value in the proposal,

Cecil Murphey, who organized and wrote the basic material,

Audrey DeLaMartre, who sat with me day after day to write and bring out the gift of this process,

Lila Empson, a fine editor who is always a pleasure, even under great pressure to meet the deadline,

My students, clients, and friends, who have understood, practiced, and internalized the Inner Eating process.

To all of you, thank you for caring and sharing!

INNER EATING

Introduction

On the icy highway, she applied the brake and the car spun forward, missing another vehicle by inches. She panicked, wrenched the wheel, and barely missed a truck coming from the opposite direction. A few seconds later she managed to stop the car. With her hands shaking and her voice trembling, she turned to her friend and said, "I'm hungry."

"Hungry? Who thinks about food at a time like this?"

"I do," she answered. "I think about food all the time."

Maybe this story seems a little exaggerated to you, but it is true to the experiences of thousands of people, male and female.

They're not kidding when they say they think about food *all* the time. They want to eat when they're happy or sad, tired or energetic, sick or well, angry or peaceful, scared or worried, busy or bored.

Through the Inner Eating process, I've worked with a variety of people who have told me about their eating habits, their attitudes, their bodies, and themselves. I've met people who

- when complimented on their figures said, "But I've got my mother's heavy thighs."
- stayed within the normal weight range but thought about eating constantly.
- looked slightly underweight but complained about feeling fat.
- constantly compared their bodies with everyone else's.
- weighed themselves as often as five times a day.

- ate huge meals in public but induced vomiting in secret.
- hated their bodies, even when they were attractive.
- said to themselves, "When I get thin, I'll . . ."
- had read a dozen diet books and been on at least as many diets but were heavier than ever.
- allowed the results from the bathroom scale to dictate whether they felt good about themselves that day.
- would eat only "good" foods while carefully avoiding "bad" and "fattening" foods.
- thought of the body as something they had but felt no real connection with it.

Did you recognize yourself in one of these statements? Perhaps several of them describe you. At the end of this Introduction you'll find a twenty-statement test to help you start becoming aware of why and how you eat.

The Inner Eating process is for people who

- have tried many diets and are still unhappy with their bodies.
- know there's something wrong with their eating but aren't sure what it is.
- don't have a healthy attitude about eating and aren't sure what to do about it.

My clients have demonstrated that they are aware that something isn't right between them and food, but they can't identify the issue and don't have the tools to deal with it—even if they could identify it.

For example, a popular misconception is that they are addicted to a particular food, often chocolate, and they fear that once they eat a bite, they won't be able to stop. The fact is, food is not addictive. However, it's possible to be allergic to a food substance and even to be preoccupied with a food or its taste. Preoccupation with a certain food is all tied up in taste and comfort, habit and guilt, and misunderstanding. No foods are forbidden to you. Barring allergic reactions, the only thing that determines what you eat is your own choice.

Are you one of those individuals who has no sense of when you're actually full? Do you know what it's like when you're hungry and when you have a bloated stomach but can't recognize anything in between?

When our bodies require nutrition, that is, fuel, we feel hunger. But other feelings and needs are experienced as hunger as well: fear, as we saw in the opening paragraph, excitement or stress, loneliness or anticipation, reward for a job well done or frustration over a job not yet done, pressure or anger, nervousness or restlessness, sadness or grief. It is interesting that both a sense of power and a sense of powerlessness are felt as hunger.

Taste is also an issue. Although it isn't an emotion, it can be an intensely pleasurable feeling that you want to sustain. So you keep eating because the food tastes so good.

Or you've learned to make food an instant problem solver. You face a dilemma. You don't know what to do, so you eat and the problem doesn't seem quite so overwhelming.

Or you eat fast! Our culture has become so preoccupied with speed that we not only eat for every reason, but we can eat faster, and more, before we're even aware of what we're doing. Whether we are in the workplace or the home, we feel deprived if we can't have something quick and easy to nibble on, just in case starvation overtakes us in the next two hours. The nibble isn't as significant in terms of volume as it is indicative of the pattern we've developed of grazing—munching our way through the day.

If you see yourself in these pictures, you may have put on weight or are afraid that you will. Maybe you're disgusted with the way your body looks. Maybe you've jumped on several diets because they promised to take the weight off without any effort on your part. Perhaps diets enabled you to avoid facing unpleasant emotions or dealing with problems that lie below the surface. Even if the diet (or diets) worked, weight loss was only temporary.

Inner Eating Isn't a Diet

Losing weight, although important, is a bonus from becoming intimately aware of your mind, body, and emotions and how they interact with your eating habits. If the purpose of Inner Eating was only to get rid of pounds, this would be a diet book, but I want something more essential for you. I want you to be able to make choices about your eating. The Inner Eating process helps you to free yourself from the tyranny of food in your life. Once you eat only to maintain your body, the weight will come off naturally. And you'll probably find that as you feel better about your body, you'll want to exercise.

The Inner Eating process doesn't tell you what to eat, how much to eat, or when to eat. You won't need to cook special foods or weigh your food or yourself. Yet it isn't easy, and it isn't magic. It will take commitment on your part. You'll learn to understand and care so much about yourself that you will invest the time and the effort to become the best you can be.

I want to talk to you as honestly and as personally as I can through printed pages. I care about you as a person, I respect you as a unique and valuable individual, and I recognize that you have your own set of reasons for eating as you do. You will learn to listen to the quiet messages that your body gives you and to respect what causes those messages—what's going on in your head that makes you want to eat or not eat.

"You know why I like Inner Eating? You accepted me for what I was right now, not where I was going to be," said Judy Brown.[1] Because I accepted her, she felt free to still her self-critical voices and accept her validity, present and future.

I developed the Inner Eating process over a period of ten years. It is a self-awareness approach that will

- show you how to free yourself from external controls.
- teach you freedom of choice about your eating.
- enable you to discover your unique eating pattern.
- guide you to recognize the reasons behind your eating.
- coach you to get in tune with your own body.
- prepare you to sense, perhaps for the first time, satisfaction and enjoyment of food.

You will also learn how to take responsibility for your eating behavior. You will

- define your present eating pattern.
- balance taste and nutrition with variety.
- achieve balance between hunger and fullness.
- listen to your body.
- learn why your fear of fat causes anxiety toward food.
- understand why you carry excess weight.

That's a lot, isn't it? And I want it all for you because it means that you will have empowered yourself to decide which habits and behaviors you want to change and which ones you want to keep. You see, the choices are not mine, not some diet plan's, not some expert's; they are yours.

Try This Test

Below are twenty statements. As you read each one, select the answer that's most often true for you: A, Always; S, Sometimes; or N, Never.

	A	S	N
1. I label food by using terms such as *fattening, nonfattening, good, bad, allowable, forbidden.*	☐	☐	☐
2. I use food as a transition. That is, I eat as I shift from one activity to the next.	☐	☐	☐
3. I weigh myself at least once a day.	☐	☐	☐
4. I need only to see or smell food to be hungry.	☐	☐	☐
5. I fear getting fat.	☐	☐	☐
6. I'm afraid to be thin.	☐	☐	☐
7. I plan my day around what or when I will eat.	☐	☐	☐
8. I constantly try not to eat but find myself nibbling throughout the day.	☐	☐	☐
9. I hate to look at my body in a mirror.	☐	☐	☐
10. When I eat at a restaurant, I select food on the basis of calories (or fat grams or other measurements).	☐	☐	☐
11. When I eat at a restaurant, the one question I do *not* ask myself is, What would I really like to eat?	☐	☐	☐
12. I eat all the food on my plate even if I don't like it or I'm full.	☐	☐	☐
13. When I overeat, I increase my exercise program.	☐	☐	☐
14. I have to eat three meals a day.	☐	☐	☐
15. I cannot tighten or contract my stomach muscles.	☐	☐	☐

16. I compare my body with others. ☐ ☐ ☐

17. I need to get on a diet plan to feel a sense of control over my eating. ☐ ☐ ☐

18. Eating or not eating is constantly on my mind. ☐ ☐ ☐

19. I hear myself saying, "When I get thin, then I'll . . ." ☐ ☐ ☐

20. Acting like a magnet, food draws me. ☐ ☐ ☐

Number of times you chose . . . . Always _____ × 3 points = _____

Number of times you chose . . . . Sometimes _____ × 2 points = _____

Number of times you chose . . . . Never _____ × 0 points = _____

TOTAL POINTS _____

If you scored at least 8 points, *Inner Eating* will definitely help you. If you scored more than 15, you *need* this book.

NOTE

1. For the most part, I use real names, not composites or disguises, in this book. These individuals have worked hard to free themselves from the bondage of food. Their names deserve to be included here, and I have used them with their permission. In some few cases, names have been fictionalized to protect privacy.

My Story

Inner Eating As It Was
Born in My Life

1

Take It from Me

America, the land of the free, yet Americans don't allow themselves freedom with food. Our food and our bodies are restricted, analyzed, weighed, and measured, and still eating for health and hunger is often *not* why we eat. That was true of me once.

"I feel fat," I said.

Actually I wasn't fat. At five three, I weighed 130 pounds, which was heavier than I wanted to be. Because weight was constantly on my mind, I could just as well have weighed 230 pounds. Although I was only in the seventh grade, I was already concerned with weight, and I wasn't remarkably different from other girls my age.

Fortunately, I had no home pressures to lose weight. (In many families the opposite is true.) Neither my father nor my mother ever indicated to me, directly or indirectly, that I should be thinner. The atmosphere in our home was supportive overall, and my parents had a strong religious commitment. That was a positive influence on us, but never a coercion. The effect was that our family didn't use tobacco or alcohol, and drugs held no appeal for us. It was a nice, small-town, idyllic, and truly happy time.

Food was the only negative in my life.

By 1962, when I had reached the seventh grade, the thin-is-in mania had become widespread in America. It was considered clever and sophisticated to say, "One can never be too thin or too rich." Fashion models were extremely thin, as were the younger film stars. Some of

Although I was only in the seventh grade, I was already concerned with weight.

the personalities who had been around for a while, like Marilyn Monroe and Jane Russell, maintained the look that made them famous, but increasingly they were becoming exceptions. Several women we knew drank a diet drink called Metrecal or chewed Ayds candies to control or lose weight.

I got caught up in the new trend, too. I was a cheerleader all through high school. Since I had lots of energy and enthusiasm, I was comfortable with cheerleading. But being watched by those crowds of people made me feel that I should be thinner. I didn't like my body and seldom felt comfortable in my clothes.

How do I lose weight? I wondered. *How do I drop these extra pounds?* I didn't know how or where to find the help I needed.

Food comforted me, diminished my anxieties, and covered any sense that I might not be doing as well as I wished.

Now, I can see clearly why I put on the pounds and why I couldn't get rid of them. Food was my companion. Food diminished my anxieties and covered any sense that I might not be doing as well as I wished.

Achievement gives me a high. I can be pretty intense about it. Everything I was involved in—sports, schoolwork, and music— became a competition. I did well, and I kept pushing myself, competing with myself.

But achieving has its downside as well, as I would learn. When I couldn't achieve weight loss, I felt like a failure. I didn't like the feeling.

I watched my father design and create a revolutionary farm building that earned him national acclaim. My mother's arena was smaller, but she was no less accomplished as a strong, soft-spoken, college-educated woman, dedicated to her profession of teaching and to her family. One year she was awarded Minnesota's Mother of the Year.

If I got stumped or felt any kind of negative feeling, I'd eat.

Following my parents' examples, I sought new challenges and pursued them single-mindedly until I conquered them. If I had a problem, if success didn't come quickly enough, if I got stumped or felt any kind of negative feeling, I'd eat.

Despite all the support at home, the achievements, and the positive experiences, I felt fat. All the time. I wanted to be thin, but I couldn't accomplish it.

When I went away to college, I gained more weight. Pictures taken then show me looking like a little football player—solid body and nicely developed muscles, certainly not the figure of the current models.

When I was nineteen, my father, a source of strong, unconditional love, died from pancreatitis. However, as a typical, stoic Swedish family, we didn't mourn excessively; we were rocks. We kept going. And I ate. When my heart hurt, I ate.

Since then I've learned that repressed emotions will find an outlet. I found mine in food. It comforted me during periods of grief, loneliness, and anxiety.

My college major was physical education and health. I challenged myself to complete the four-year degree program in three years. My adviser said, "You can't do it in three years." But I knew I could find a way. During those three years on my self-designed treadmill, I was preoccupied with my weight and fought to keep the same number in the center of my scale's dial.

I wasn't aware that I had made eating a must-do activity, a duty no different from studying or getting an *A* or striving for any other achievement. I certainly didn't think of it as taking care of my body. But I was becoming aware of my weight and the challenge to get rid of all that I considered excessive.

It seemed natural and logical to me that I could get rid of the weight by setting up a program and working hard at it the way I had with my education programs and every other challenge in my life. That approach had always paid off before. But to my dismay and utter confusion, it didn't work. This was something I couldn't accomplish with determination. Obviously it would take something else, but I had no idea what. The problem plagued me from college to my teaching career.

Betty Litten, a coteacher and friend, was also concerned about the fat-thin problem, but she managed to stay thinner than I. To stay at her predetermined weight, Betty would cut her food intake way back during the week—famine. Then came the weekend, and by noon Saturday she had blown it—feast. Monday, she would be back in school, determined to adhere to her diet—famine again.

One of the things that I enjoyed about Betty was her ability to identify, feel, and express her emotions. That ability was a gift that our friendship affirmed in me. It was a pleasure, a relief, to acknowledge that I felt frustration, grief, anxiety, and doubt as well as joy, excitement, playfulness, and peace. It was all part of my learning to feel like a whole person.

Learning to feel comfortable with having emotions didn't do anything to help me combat my weight, however. Still unaware of my

I've learned that repressed emotions will find an outlet. I found mine in food. It comforted me during periods of grief, loneliness, and anxiety.

I wasn't aware that I had made eating a must-do activity, a duty no different from studying or getting an A or any striving for other achievement.

Still unaware of my motives, whenever I encountered frustration or stress, I ate.

motives, whenever I encountered frustration or stress, I ate. I thought of food in terms of what it would do for my body size, nothing else. Instead of eating to care for my body, I ate to achieve the physical image I wanted, just like Betty did.

We were caught up in a cycle in which we'd do well at school, sometimes for as long as three weeks, and then we'd rebel against the restrictions of our current diets and eat according to our appetites and urges. We destroyed our diets, felt guilty, and vowed to try even harder.

Of course, because we couldn't stay on any diet, we assumed we lacked strength of mind. We never dreamed that we were just fine in the willpower department, and that our struggle had nothing whatever to do with our powers of resolve. So, we continued to live that way—never getting too heavy and never, never getting thin enough.

About that time, some of my students—in those days, only girls seemed aware of a weight problem—came to me and asked, "How can I lose weight?" We had good conversations, and they were open with me. I really cared about them and respected their desire to feel good about themselves. As a conscientious physical education teacher, I collected the available information and put them on balanced diets.

Unfortunately, they had three major complaints—and they sounded like my own:

- ▪ "I'm hungry all the time."
- ▪ "I keep wanting to eat more."
- ▪ "I think about my weight and food all the time."

Out of my concern for the girls, I started writing down rules for them to make dieting easier, such as which foods to eat, which ones to avoid, and how much to eat. Like everyone else, I prescribed restrictions for weight loss. With my background in health and nutrition, I never suggested anything extremely low in calories. Mostly I laid out a list of do's and don'ts.

But the diets weren't enough. Restrictions and nutrition information weren't enough.

The girls followed rules, but they were my rules. Those rules didn't help them learn how to figure out what felt right for their bodies.

Then I realized something that one day would be important in my Inner Eating process. The girls followed rules, but they were *my* rules. Those rules didn't help them learn how to figure out what felt right for their bodies. In fact, their knowledge of their bodies was generally superficial, based on textbook material.

Many of them could devour ten cookies or an entire box, but they couldn't eat just *one* cookie. So they binged or fasted. And I would do the same things.

They told me how they felt after bingeing, using words like *yucky, stuffed, nauseated,* and *uncomfortable.* They still had no sense that anything was wrong with restrictions, and they blamed themselves for their lack of willpower.

About that time the diet craze consumed the United States. Every magazine and newspaper promised schemes to lose weight. New diet books appeared monthly. If one diet didn't work, next week there would be another one. It became a game, a very sad game, to find the magic solution in someone's diet plan. So I learned all about diets, and I tried several.

Soon thereafter I married Jon Billigmeier, and it wasn't long before I noticed his eating pattern. Jon would sit down, eat what he wanted, and then stop eating, relax, and chat with me until I was finished. He never ate more or less than he wanted.

When he finished eating, the meal was over for him. That is, he didn't go from the table to a bowl of candy or an extra nibble of dessert; he'd go on to other things. For Jon, the thought of food didn't carry over into any other activity. He wasn't filling his mind with thoughts of what he would eat for the next meal, the next hour, or the next day.

For Jon, the thought of food didn't carry over into any other activity. He wasn't filling his mind with thoughts of what he would eat for the next meal, the next hour, or the next day.

Of course, Jon didn't spend much of his day dealing with food in one way or another: shopping, budgeting, planning meals, cooking meals, putting food away, and cleaning up the kitchen. Most people who are responsible for making the household's meals become preoccupied with food because it's necessary to keep planning ahead. These people, men and women alike, often lose the ability to interpret the messages their bodies are sending, reading all signals as hunger because of the prominent role food plays in their lives. I'll talk about that problem, the inability to interpret your body's messages and some of the reasons for it, later.

Jon's daily eating pattern was different from mine. If you'll look at the illustration of our eating patterns at the time, you'll notice a lot of circles beneath our names. (See 1-A.) Each circle represents a time that we ate, an eating occasion. A big circle is a large amount, usually a meal, and a small circle is a snack or a nibble. It's obvious that I was the one preoccupied with food.

My eating circles are connected because food never really left my mind. I went from eating to thinking about eating to eating continuously. As I said above, Jon's eating experiences were separated by periods in which he didn't think about food.

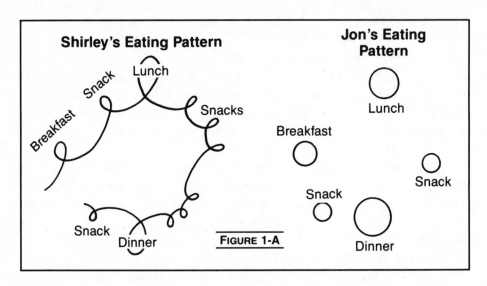

Shirley's Eating Pattern

Breakfast
Snack
Lunch
Snacks
Snack
Dinner

Jon's Eating Pattern

Lunch
Breakfast
Snack
Snack
Dinner

FIGURE 1-A

One day when we went to a restaurant, Jon opened the menu, looked it over, and made his selection.

When he put his menu down, I asked something that had been bothering me for a long time. "Do you think about food? Do you think about your weight? Do you ever weigh yourself?"

"Do you think about food? Do you think about your weight? Do you ever weigh yourself?"

"Not much," he said with a quizzical smile, ready to dismiss the subject. Food apparently wasn't that important to him.

"Wait," I said, puzzled by his attitude. "How can you be so unconcerned about food? You eat and it's over? You don't think about food again?"

He thought for a minute before he answered. "I guess that about covers it. Until I'm hungry again, that is."

At first I didn't believe him. My friends and I thought about food, talked about food, ate, dieted, planned menus, and talked some more about food. It was our major topic of conversation.

Food was our major topic of conversation.

"I eat when I'm hungry, and I enjoy the food it takes to satisfy that hunger," Jon said, "but that's all. My weight's not much different from when I graduated from high school."

From then on, I carefully watched Jon's behavior. Unlike my friends and I, Jon did not put off eating as long as he could each morning. Not Jon.

"I'm hungry," he'd say, minutes after getting out of bed.

"Can't you wait?"

"Sure I could," he'd answer. "But I'm hungry now."

Hungry? What does hunger have to do with it? I wondered.

So Jon had breakfast as soon as he could each morning. Later he'd have lunch, something light around five-thirty, and a meal around seven, followed by cookies and milk in the evening.

Jon ate five times a day. That was his pattern. But he thought little about food at other times. Did I ever envy him! And why shouldn't I?

- He was never on a diet.
- He didn't think about his weight.
- He wasn't burdened with a heavy exercise program, yet he maintained his preferred weight.

That's what I want, I thought. *That's the goal I want to achieve with my eating.*

So, still the compulsive achiever with a new challenge, I determined that I would discover why Jon was the way he was. Then I would adapt to that way. I was still looking for an external solution for my internal relationship with food.

I was still looking for an external solution for my internal relationship with food.

"How do I learn to eat like you, Jon?" I asked him.

"I don't know," he said and shook his head at my question.

He really didn't know, and he couldn't understand my preoccupation with the issue. He simply didn't think that much about food or weight or diet.

About that time I began what eventually would become a journal. Every time I thought about weight, I'd write it down. Sometimes I had only questions:

Is it just a matter of eating so many calories? Is that it? Yet Jon never asks himself how many calories he's eating. He really doesn't care about calories. No, that's not it. But if it's not, then what is?

Whenever I tried to work with calories, and that's what most diets are based on, it always became a numbers game. As soon as I went over the magic limit, I had blown it. I had failed more than the diet; I was a failure in being a good person, in trying to be strong, and in living up to my ideals.

I was dealing with something entirely different from my education and background. Everything in my experience had said that the more precisely I worked, the better I did. However, my eating habits didn't seem to understand those rules. The more precise I became, the less control I seemed to have over my eating.

The more precise I became, the less control I seemed to have over my eating.

Still, I went back to the calories, because that's all I knew. I tried counting and limiting and exchanging calories. I lost weight—temporarily. As long as I deprived—punished—myself, I could lose. As soon as I relaxed—rebelled, I called it—the weight crept back on, with an extra pound or two.

I enrolled at a local diet center and lost fifteen pounds. Yet my eating and thought processes were still the same. Nothing had changed, really.

That's not quite true. I did have one new thing—a tormenting worry. I feared that my weight would start climbing upward again. Sure, I had lost the weight, but what if it came back, with an extra five pounds? Would I have to go on another diet? I hadn't solved any problem for myself. I didn't know what to do about my weight. Losing weight hadn't helped. If anything, dieting made the problem worse.

Losing weight hadn't helped. If anything, dieting made the problem worse.

At the same time, I felt compelled to go on another diet. I wanted to do it again. I wanted something external, some control out there, to tell me what to do and when and how.

Then a little answering voice began inside me:

I don't want to be dependent on outside controls.

I don't want to feel addicted to diets.

I want to enjoy food without being controlled by it.

I want more than weight loss; I want the kind of freedom with food that Jon has.

Maybe nutrition is the answer, I thought. *Maybe if I cut out sugar and white flour, that might work.* So I tried it, even though Jon wasn't concerned about such trivialities. Our food may have been more nutritious, but that wasn't the answer. I still overate.

I kept trying new systems. I *had* to find one that worked. Each time I went on a new diet, I assured myself that this would be the definitive

Each time I went on a new diet, I assured myself that this would be the definitive one, the successful one.

one, the successful one. No matter what it was called or how the origi- nator had set it up, soon it seemed just like all the other diets I had been on before. The results were far from satisfactory.

Finally, I asked myself, *Shirley, what's the real problem?*

"I don't know," I answered.

Where will it end?

"I don't know," I answered.

When you begin eating, there's no problem. You just don't know how to end it.

"I know. I can't seem to stop—whether it's actually eating or just thinking about it."

You don't end. You begin eating and just keep on.

I sat with my chin on my hand and thought about the conversation I'd just had with myself. I noticed that two ideas were repeated— *beginning* and *ending*—and I wondered about their significance. Be- ginning and ending.

How do I begin to eat? How do I end a meal? I thought. Maybe that was part of the problem because I never started a meal, finished it, and then moved on to something else. I started eating in the morning, and one eating occasion ran into the next, either with actual eating or with thinking about or planning for food. I didn't end a meal when I chose, either. My ending was determined by how much food was on my plate; I kept eating until my plate was clean. My eating process seemed to have no end.

I never started a meal, finished it, and then moved on to something else.

A few days later I wrote in my journal:

Beginning and ending. What does that mean?

I was working my way out of the diet mentality, and I didn't want to go back. I had to move beyond those mechanical, rigid, external boundaries.

Where are all these issues about food coming from? I wondered. *Why do I think about food all day long? If counting calories isn't the answer, what is? Self-discipline? No, that can't be the solution. Look at Jon. He doesn't use willpower. He simply stops because he's had enough. But how do I know when I've had enough? I don't know. Jon must have something inside him that I lack—some sense of internal boundaries.*

If counting calories isn't the answer, what is?

That's it! My eyes flew open wide. *Internal boundaries!*

I hadn't yet developed a sense of internal limits for my eating. That's why I continued to search for an external limitation—a diet, a rule, something to set the limits for me. Jon set his own. I needed to learn to set my own. But how?

One day I realized something else about food. It was one of those significant moments that changed my entire way of looking at food. Eating was an *activity* for me. An event. Even a challenge. It was something I *did* the way I would tackle any other challenge.

Although I had given myself plenty of negative feedback for overeating, I had no positive feelings about eating, at all.

For me, that insight was like a brilliant light in a dim room. Eating had become something I did purposefully. It was not an aspect of enjoying life or a means of taking care of my body. I never felt free just to eat. It had to have a purpose. My eating or not eating was to attain a certain body size, not simply to savor the food in front of me. Although I had given myself plenty of negative feedback for overeating, I had no positive feelings about eating.

I was used to attaining positive results in the other areas of my life. Therefore, I was sure that somewhere, somehow, I would find an answer so I could feel positive about my eating and about my body.

As soon as I started putting restrictions on what I could eat, I set myself up to fail.

Then came another insight. As soon as I started putting restrictions on *what* I could eat, I set myself up to fail. If I decided what I *had* to eat, I wouldn't want those foods. If I went the other way and *restricted* my diet and made out a list of forbidden foods, I'd find myself yearning for them. Childish, I know, but predictably human.

At that point I encountered the book *The Marshall Plan for Lifelong Weight Control.* I liked Edward Marshall's advice, which was built around one concept: choose whatever you want to eat, but eat only when you're hungry.

Aha, I thought, *this is a start. I'll eat only when I'm hungry.* I still wasn't sure how to know when I was hungry, but I was willing to give it a try.

For the first time since seventh grade I had a glimpse of freedom—it was only for a brief moment—yet I knew Marshall was moving in the right direction.

With that new concept, I was launched in a direction that ultimately would prove fruitful. I brought back into the house all the foods that I had restricted earlier. However, my background nagged, *But, Shirley, too much sugar and fat is bad for you. You need to put nutrition into your diet.*

So I combined Dr. Marshall's information with everything I knew about nutrition, exercise, and weight loss. I sensed that I was getting closer to my answer. Still being the achiever, I plunged into the project. The answer for me, I knew, lay in establishing my internal boundary of hunger, and I had to figure it out for myself.

In our home, I had designed a large room just for exercise classes. Since I was no longer teaching at a junior high school, I invited friends to come in for free lessons to teach them about fitness and eating. In return, I asked them for their honest feedback. Later I turned it into a full-fledged business called the Fitness Forum. I became a consultant on fitness, body image, and weight control.

I asked the volunteers to try eating only when they were hungry and let me know how it worked. It worked well—for about two weeks. But then they began to eat when they weren't hungry, and they felt guilty about it. Then they were back to the

diet mentality, which led to - - - - - - - - - - - - - - ->
failure, which led to - - - - - - - - - - - - - - - - - ->
guilt, which led to ->
                                        another diet.

Back to the drawing board.

Even though eating only when hungry wasn't the whole solution, I felt that it was the right place to start, so I began to concentrate on the word *hunger* as a body signal. Hunger means the body needs food. *Could that pose a problem?* I wondered.

I considered what it would be like if I worked in an office and couldn't always eat whenever I wanted to. If I eat only when I'm hungry, what happens when noon comes and my stomach says it doesn't want food? Should I go out with the others and eat anyway? Or stay at my desk and not eat? If I don't eat, in an hour I know I'm going to be hungry. Then lunch hour will be over, and I don't like to eat alone.

Or suppose I'm sitting in an important business meeting and I get hungry. I can't eat there and then, and the meeting will run for at least another hour. If I'm hungry and I can't eat, has the plan failed?

No, it was apparent that hunger alone wasn't the entire answer.

But wait a minute. It's a process. It doesn't mean that I must eat immediately or that I have to fill the tank full every time, does it? The amount I eat can vary according to occasion and need. For example, I

The answer for me, I knew, lay in establishing my internal boundary of hunger, and I had to figure it out for myself.

If I eat only when I'm hungry, what happens when noon comes and my stomach says it doesn't want food?

It's a process. . . . The amount I eat can vary according to occasion and need.

can eat a light meal when I'm not particularly hungry and then have a snack later at a coffee break. If I'm not urgently hungry then I can choose to postpone eating until after work.

While I was working on this concept, I attended a workshop in California in which one leader urged participants to "always have food with you, so that whenever you get hungry, you can feed that hunger." Each day, she said, she prepared little packages of food. If she was in a meeting and felt hungry, she could eat.

That might work, I thought, *in a meeting about eating issues. But it would be inappropriate and awkward in a boardroom or a sales meeting to have people pull out little packets of food and nibble.*

Yet the principle was right—eat only when hungry. I just had to figure out how to make it work in our society.

People need guidelines, not external controls.

From that point I was convinced that laying down strict rules wasn't the answer. People need guidelines, not external controls. My experience with diets had shown me that external controls, boundaries, will work only for a while. I wanted to offer the kind of help that would enable people to make choices for themselves, to create internal boundaries.

I visualized a circle representing and containing each eating occasion.

That's when I moved on to the next step in developing my process. By thinking again of beginning and ending, I visualized a circle representing and containing each eating occasion. The idea felt right as a tool for creating the boundaries I sought.

A circle is an area of containment, of completeness, of wholeness. Everything you have eaten on that occasion goes into the circle, and when you complete the circle, you have created your boundary for the occasion. (In the next chapter I will deal with this idea more fully.)

All the while I worked with circles, I read current research material about diet and health. A few voices were beginning to speak out against restrictive diets. Other researchers were turning their attention to physical health and writing about how to achieve it. The body needs variety, they were saying. One expert advocated six small meals instead of three large ones. I continued monitoring myself and my volunteers, keeping track of research, and writing frequently about feelings and thoughts. Essentially, that's how Inner Eating began.

Inner Eating is a holistic process that is not built around structure, steps, and rules.

Inner Eating is a holistic process that is not built around structure, steps, and rules. It is a personal encounter process that's similar to peeling an artichoke. Each artichoke leaf represents an issue attached to the act of eating that has nothing to do with the act of eating. Little by little each person peels away his or her leaves, one by one strips them through the teeth to get nourishment from them, and throws them away. When at last the heart of the artichoke is reached, what is revealed is eating for enjoyment and nutrition without fear of fat.

In the following chapters I'll show you how to integrate the principles that grew out of the eat-only-when-you're-hungry concept into your lifestyle. I include gentle reminders called Note to Myself to help you implement the Inner Eating process. I also use diagrams to give you a clearer picture of each part of the process.

At the end of each chapter, you'll find Steps to Build On, suggestions for things you can do to work through the process of Inner Eating.

I also recommend that you keep a journal. It helps you reveal your inner chatter and then deal with it, it helps you keep track of and analyze the events and feelings—past and present—that fuel your eating practices, and it offers you a place to cheer yourself on.

┌─ **NOTE TO MYSELF** ──────────────────┐
│ *I respect myself as I am right now. I respect my* │
│ *body as it is right now.* │
└──┘

I used the word *respect* because you might find it difficult to say that you *like* yourself or your body right now. Often people are afraid to accept or like their bodies because they fear that if they do, they will lose their drive for improvement. But the opposite of liking your body is disliking it, and if you dislike your body, you're inclined to punish it. You've been punishing it because you haven't respected it. Now you need to respect your body to get started, and that respect will be built upon throughout the Inner Eating process. In your relationship with yourself, as with other people, you are free to like or dislike various parts of your physical self. But just as you can achieve harmony with other people only through mutual respect, so you must respect yourself to be in harmony with yourself.

Just as you can achieve harmony with other people only through mutual respect, so you must respect yourself to be in harmony with yourself.

CHAPTER SUMMARY

Emotions and feelings are essential to make you feel whole. Willpower isn't enough to cause you to lose weight and keep it off. External controls, like restrictive diets, may work briefly, but they don't continue to be effective because your relationship with food is internal and unique. An eating occasion has a beginning and an ending, and it can be defined as contained in a circle. You need to create eating boundaries for yourself and not depend on external authority. Respecting yourself is a beginning.

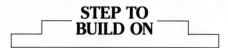

STEP TO
BUILD ON

1. Write down the Note to Myself from this chapter. Do the same with each chapter as you complete it. Keep them where you'll see them regularly, on your mirror, refrigerator, desk, or perhaps the dashboard of your car.

Inner Eating Process

2

Creating Boundaries

"You'd have to describe me as a Pac-Man eater," Jackie Singer said when we first talked about circles. Like the character in the video game, Jackie nibbled her way through the entire day.

"Even so, I'd like you to keep track of each act of eating," I told her. "Think of it this way: each circle you draw represents each eating session."

"If I did that, I'd have thirty circles," she said. "Maybe more."

"I'm not concerned about the number of circles. I won't condemn you or tell you that you have too many circles. Eating is an individual thing, not a pass-fail assignment," I assured her. "Don't put it off; start where you are right now. You'll be pleasantly surprised at what this tool helps you to see about your eating pattern."

Jackie's smile reflected her reservations about this exercise, but she agreed to do it.

"It will give you a visual means to see how you eat," I told her. "Each time you begin an eating occasion, whether it's a couple of nuts as you pass the dish in the living room or a cookie eaten while you stand looking out the window or a sit-down meal, the circle begins. When you stop eating, the circle closes. Your circle will isolate and make visible each eating occasion."

By drawing circles on a piece of paper to isolate and represent each eating occasion, you make visible your eating pattern. Once you can see your pattern, you can evaluate it for yourself and make an

"Each time you begin an eating occasion, whether it's a couple of nuts as you pass the dish in the living room or a cookie eaten while you stand looking out the window or a sit-down meal, the circle begins. When you stop eating, the circle closes."

informed decision about whether you need to change it and how.

People who deal with food all day long—people in the restaurant business, grocers, food vendors and preparers, and homemakers—say that focusing so much on food is a problem. It certainly can be a factor, I agree. But the fact remains that *the act of eating creates the problem.* Thinking about food can be a trigger, but it has no calories.

Calories don't affect the body unless they're ingested, and most people are unaware of what, how, and when they eat. Before you can do anything to change your eating habits, you need to understand and acknowledge your particular eating pattern.

As I developed my Inner Eating process over the years, I tried several ways to help clients understand their eating patterns and what they mean. Circles proved to be the most helpful tool for people to work with. I hope you will use this method to create boundaries for your eating pattern.

Boundaries set limits. We put boundaries between our personalities and others' to help us define ourselves. We put boundaries between our emotions and others' to be responsible for how we feel. We even set boundaries around what fashions we choose to wear so we're not victims of every passing fashion fad. Boundaries are not walls; they are limits we choose. Flexibility and wisdom are essential for boundary maintenance.

It's possible to set boundaries so rigidly that nothing can change them. An example of a too-rigid food boundary might be, "I *must* clean my plate." Parents set that kind of boundary for young children out of concern for their health, not realizing that children have good food sense, even if parents can't see it. Then health and obedience and parental control get confused in the child's mind while he or she is still too young to have a good sense of self, and circumstances set rigid eating boundaries that are no longer appropriate.

On the other hand, boundaries that are too flexible or weak can't withstand temptation, such as television and magazine ads for food or another person urging, "Aw, c'mon, just taste it." "Have another little helping; it won't hurt you." "Have a dish of ice cream with me; keep me company."

Having no boundaries or allowing circumstances to set boundaries for you can cause you to overeat or undereat and lose sight of the goal you have set for yourself. Boundaries that are firm but not rigid give you strength to maintain your choices and decisions.

Boundaries are not walls; they are limits we choose.

Having no boundaries or allowing circumstances to set boundaries for you can cause you to overeat or undereat and lose sight of the goal you have set for yourself.

In my opinion, people have gravitated toward diets as a means of weight control because their boundaries have not been established. Also, they don't realize that they have the option of creating their own boundaries.

The boundaries I'm asking you to depict are choices you make freely. They're not restrictive, only descriptive. The boundary is represented by a circle, and each eating experience is within the circle. You begin the circle each time you begin eating, and you close it when you end that eating occasion, whether it's a brownie or a banquet. Vary the size of your circles to indicate the amount of intake—a banquet is a bigger circle than a brownie. A candy bar is a small circle. Milk and cookies indicate a small circle. Soup, sandwich, and coffee call for a slightly bigger circle. A full dinner is an even bigger circle. Two plates full at a buffet dinner mean a bi-i-ig circle.

By drawing appropriate-sized circles in a notebook each day, you can see the way you eat, and each eating occasion is acknowledged without prejudice. You have a record showing that *all* eating counts as food intake, including the little snacks and nibbles.

There are a couple different ways to place the circles on the paper each day. In this book, I will place them as if they were on a clock indicating the approximate time the food was eaten. (See 2-A.)

Vary the size of your circles to indicate the amount of intake—a banquet is a bigger circle than a brownie.

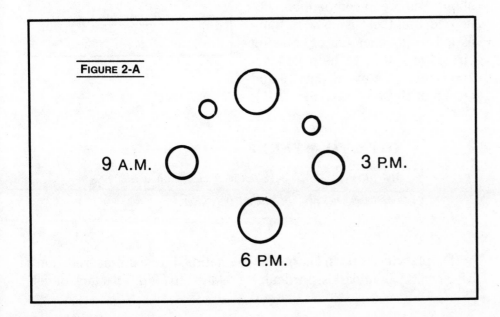

FIGURE 2-A

9 A.M.　　　3 P.M.

6 P.M.

One client preferred to place the circles in a straight line and periodically place a time on the line. (See 2-B.)

He said he ate many times during the day and into the night. He said he would need both an A.M. clock and a P.M. clock for each day so his eating circles wouldn't keep overlapping! Choose what works best for you.

You can see how weekdays and weekends differ, how daytime and evening differ. Then if you feel you want to lose weight or gain weight, you will have a visual guide to work with.

There is no such thing as failure in Inner Eating.

When I said that each eating occasion is acknowledged without prejudice, that was both a statement of fact and a plea. Please, don't condemn yourself for the number and size of your circles. That's *not* what Inner Eating is about. You are in competition with no one, and there is no such thing as failure in Inner Eating. Making circles is a tool to help you acknowledge your eating pattern and change it *if you choose.* (See 2-C.)

6 A.M. ◯

◯

◯

12 NOON ◯

◯

3 P.M. ◯

◯

◯

6 P.M. ◯

FIGURE 2-B

NOTE TO MYSELF

Each time I eat I will draw a circle on a piece of paper to represent that eating occasion.

People who aren't in charge of their eating, I have discovered, don't have healthy boundaries, particularly relating to food. That lack of definition acts like internal smog that prevents a clear view of their eating patterns and motivations. Sometimes the smog is only a moderate haze, such as that over a lake on a summer morning, but often it's as thick and choking as a Los Angeles temperature inversion smog with the same potential for blocking out the sunlight of clear thinking. Usually the people who are smogged in think about food and/ or eat all day long. (See 2-D.)

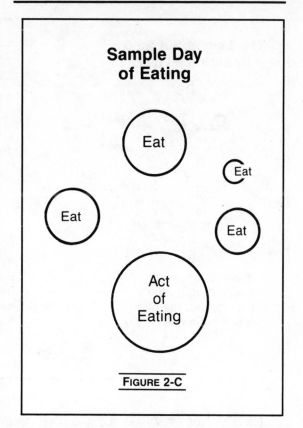

Sample Day of Eating

Eat

Eat

Eat

Eat

Act
of
Eating

FIGURE 2-C

But getting back to Jackie's story, it wasn't easy for her to draw all those circles, admitting that she ate constantly, but she followed through. Her awareness of her eating pattern was vague, and despite calling herself a Pac-Man eater, she was still amazed at how many times a day she put food into her body. Not a lot of food each time, but the small circles added up to a considerable quantity.

The pattern of the circles helped her see that the real Pac-Man mentality kicked in late in the afternoon. She started with snacks and just kept going until bedtime. Then she felt stuffed and guilty for allowing herself to get that way (See 2-E).

─**NOTE TO MYSELF**─

Becoming aware of my eating pattern will help me understand what I'm doing.

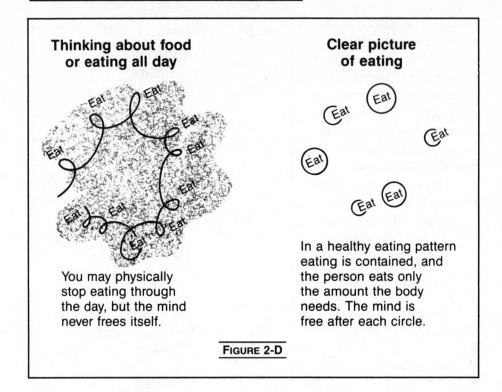

Thinking about food or eating all day

You may physically stop eating through the day, but the mind never frees itself.

Clear picture of eating

In a healthy eating pattern eating is contained, and the person eats only the amount the body needs. The mind is free after each circle.

FIGURE 2-D

(NOTE: Not everyone feels stuffed or even guilty about constant snacking at a particular time of day or all day. Some people just do it. It isn't until they work with the circles for a while that they understand the consequences of what seemed like just a comfortable indulgence. They develop "love handles" or their belts get tighter, and they decide to take off a couple of pounds. The value of using the circles for them is that once they see the eating pattern and know *why* they gained weight, they can choose to change the pattern and be rid of the love-handle problem.)

Later Jackie said, "I ate quickly, with no thought about how fast I was eating or how much I was actually putting into my body."

Now she prepares about half what she used to eat, and she's learned what it feels like to reach the balance point—she calls it the comfort zone—where she has had just enough but not too much.

"I don't waste my taste buds on food I don't like anymore. I used to feel like Pac-Man as I chomped my way through food. Now I eat like a lady. I enjoy my food without that uncomfortable sense of being stuffed, and I don't feel guilty. I used to yo-yo through diets between 110 and 130 pounds. I've stayed at 115 to 118 since I've used Inner Eating."

It isn't unusual for people to resist drawing the circles, feeling they can do the rest of the process without them. That response is so predictable, in fact, that I've developed four reasons for the wisdom of their use.

First, by drawing each circle, you own—admit, accept—where you are right now with the eating you are doing today. It's not guesswork, and it's a way to help you be honest with yourself. By seeing a boundary, eventually you will start to internalize it, and it will be yours.

By seeing a boundary, eventually you will start to internalize it, and it will be yours.

Making a commitment to work with the circles, then, is often a stumbling block. I recall when Chip Fisher talked to me about his eating. "When my life calms down, I can get on a good nutrition program."

"Why wait?" I asked. "You're an active man who loves having a lot of things happening in your life. That may never change. Own where you are now. Acknowledge it with a circle each time you eat. That's how you start."

Second, by drawing the circles, you can see how *often* you eat. Nibblers, tasters, and grazers especially need to be aware of this. You may eat a spoonful of ice cream or two potato chips or five grapes, but they still count. Because they're such small amounts, you may not be aware of your total consumption.

You may not be aware of your total consumption.

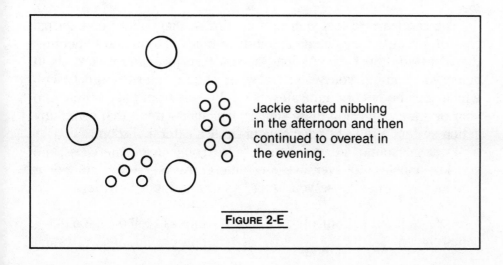

Jackie started nibbling in the afternoon and then continued to overeat in the evening.

FIGURE 2-E

Third, drawing circles is the first big step toward giving you the freedom to think about things other than food between meals.

In addition to creating a beginning and an ending for each act of eating, you need to create a beginning and an ending for your thoughts about eating. Like many other people, you may have a constant chatter going on inside your head. (The word *chatter* works for me because I have a full-blown conversation going on in my head. For others, it may be more like a buzz of remembered voices that exists at a subliminal or subconscious level.) Once you begin taking charge of your eating occasions, your other activities won't be blurred with chatter or buzz—that preoccupation with eating.

Once you begin taking charge of your eating occasions, your other activities won't be blurred with chatter or buzz—that preoccupation with eating.

One client was puzzled by my use of the word *chatter*. She listened, frowning thoughtfully. I thought she simply didn't understand, so I tried again to make myself clear. Suddenly her face lit with understanding. She told me that she wondered why she didn't have chatter or even a buzz of voices going on in her head. There was nothing, she said, and that confused her until she realized that the voices were blanketed by years of habitual behavior. When she was younger, she had felt the guilt, the defiance, and the challenging of the voices. But she no longer heard the chatter. As she worked with the circles and the rest of the Inner Eating process, she worked through that blanket to the voices and the issues hidden beneath it.

Fourth, drawing circles helps you clarify your internal boundaries. Don't let that thought overwhelm you; you already possess these self-restraints. *I want to teach you how to be aware of them and to activate them.*

As long as you turn to external controls to guide your eating, you won't feel your natural internal signals with which your body communicates its food needs from your stomach to your brain.

You can learn to feel your internal limits. Diets offer you external controls because they dictate amounts or kinds of food and sometimes the times you must eat. As long as you turn to external controls to guide your eating, you won't feel your natural internal signals with which your body communicates its food needs from your stomach to your brain. By ignoring these signals, you short-circuit that communication system and fight against your body's natural wisdom.

Does this sound like you? You were hard on yourself, merciless, and you felt hopeless to ever live any differently. When you stuffed or binged, you turned loose your guilt feelings and inner chatter.

- ▪ You felt out of control: "Oh, well, as long as I fell off the diet anyway."

- You beat yourself up with guilty notions: "If I wasn't so weak, I wouldn't have given in and eaten that."
- You hated yourself for being weak, for not being strong enough to resist: "I failed again. I'm a failure. Why can't I leave that food alone? What's wrong with me?"

As the pounds began to creep back on, you punished or disciplined yourself by going on another diet.

But that's past now. You don't have to go through that self-defeating process anymore. Using the tools of Inner Eating, you will develop inner boundaries and understanding.

You will

- understand how eating has affected your life.
- have energy through the day because you've listened to your body's signals and nourished it when it called for food.
- be at peace with your body and with each circle of eating.
- be free of diet and food bondage.

You will no longer feel obliged to think of yourself as

- fat or thin, but as a unique and valuable person.
- one who's imprisoned by an uncontrollable appetite.

You don't have to go through that self-defeating process anymore.

——————————— □ ———————————

Consider this.

1. Without using inner boundaries, *you've probably been living wholly or partially by someone else's rules for your body.* The rules may have been given by honest, well-intentioned people, but they are denying ownership of your act of eating.

2. Without using inner boundaries, *you fear food's ability to sabotage your choices.* When food is available, you go through all kinds of turmoil: "If I eat this, I'll gain weight." "If people see I have food in my desk, what will they think?" "If I pass it up, I'll miss out." "It smells too good to resist."

3. Without using inner boundaries, *you let feelings make the choice for you.* "I know what they're thinking, and I'm going to eat anyway." "I'm so happy/sad/nervous/excited; if I don't eat something, I'll burst."

You've probably been living wholly or partially by someone else's rules for your body.

You let feelings make the choice for you.

4. Without using inner boundaries, *you live in a food smog*. This smog of eating or thinking about eating clouds over and wreaths around all your day's activities. You're robbed of your pleasures, even the pleasure of eating.

You ignore internal signals.

5. Without using inner boundaries, *you ignore internal signals.* Linda Kemp loved bread, especially freshly baked bread. Whenever Linda and her husband went to her favorite restaurant, she would devour an entire basket of French bread while waiting for her entree. Usually she called for a second basket and finished that off, too.

By the time her food arrived, she was quite full. Linda didn't know she was so full, because she didn't know how to rely on her internal signals. She could no longer remember what her internal signals for empty and full felt like, let alone the subtle degrees in between. So when the waiter brought her meal, she did what she always did; she ate the entire meal, leaving only a clean plate.

For Linda, closing the circle of a fine meal meant physically leaving the restaurant. It didn't occur to her that she could have closed that particular circle with just the bread and balanced out other nutritional needs at the next meal.

One circle can't fix or override another circle.

One circle can't fix or override another circle. The body needs only so much food. If Linda chooses to fill up on bread, she can't erase that choice by eating a nutritious meal. (See 2-F.) For Linda, accepting the choices she'd made and knowing that she could choose differently next time were helpful.

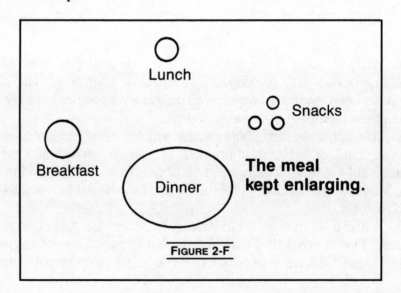

FIGURE 2-F

Think about breakfast. Each morning you probably leave for work, get the children off to school, or hurry into some other activity. That activity automatically creates an ending to breakfast.

When you put the first bite of food into your mouth, that starts breakfast. In the same way, the last bite ends breakfast. One circle is complete—probably one of several for the day. (I know this sounds oversimplified, but bear with me.)

As you have read, Linda had a pattern of overeating. Jackie had a pattern of nibbling—Chris had yet another pattern. She had been a flight attendant for ten years. In the beginning of her employment, she had to weigh in once a month. For Chris, weight was a critical issue. She wasn't overweight—although she had been once—but she felt she was fat and lived with the fear that her weight could get out of control again. Feeling that she was fat affected her attitude toward herself as much as actually being fat.

Each month Chris faced the official scale. "On the day of my weighing," she said, "I would take off my watch and shed my jewelry. I became preoccupied with my weight. I weighed myself every morning and again at night. If the dial went up as much as a pound, my mood changed for the rest of the day. I could go in feeling wonderful and end up ruining a good day. If I had gained, I would declare a diet day—a one-day fast. I was afraid that if I started something, I wouldn't be able to stop."

Chris decided to have one daily meal, in the evening, but actually she nibbled periodically throughout the day without realizing it. She was employing that strange twist of mind called eating-to-not-eat. Then when she got home and ate dinner, she kept on eating, bingeing, knowing that she would diet the next day. So her no-eating pattern developed.

Because of this overriding fear, Chris's circles eventually dwindled to just one. Her diagram looked like this. (See 2-G.) Her weight didn't go up and down, but she thought about food all the time.

Like Chris, a number of people have chosen to eat one meal at night as a means of weight control. In the words of one fitness expert:

> That's the worst way to eat for anyone trying to reduce body fat. Large meals call up large amounts of insulin, and insulin encourages calories to be stored as fat rather than burned. Worse yet, large meals tend to leave one feeling drowsy, and hence uninclined to do much more than sink into the nearest sofa.[1]

People may say, "I'm inclined to be fat so I'll just eat one meal in the evening to control my weight," yet the opposite may be happening—"I eat only in the evening; therefore, I will be fat." These people could be

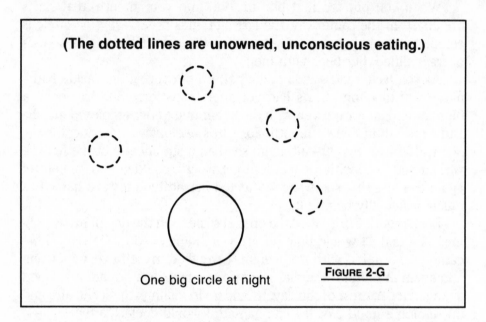

(The dotted lines are unowned, unconscious eating.)

One big circle at night

FIGURE 2-G

sabotaging themselves and their metabolism. The Inner Eating process gives these individuals the tools and knowledge to work with their bodies, instead of against them.

———————————— □ ————————————

I've shown you the eating patterns of three individuals. Although each one drew a different set of circles, they shared at least three common problems with eating.

- They had no structure.
  - They had no internal control.
    - They didn't understand their relationship to food until they went through this simple procedure of defining their eating patterns.

People are drawn to diets because diets give them external controls and feelings of safety. When they go off those controls, they enter a nightmare world called Fat Attack Land, where fat and food lurk to attack. Consequently, they want to run right back to the safety of Diet Land.

The best way to keep track of your eating is to carry a piece of paper in your pocket and record each time you pop anything into your mouth. Vary the size of the circle to represent the volume: some grapes, a donut, a cracker, coffee with a sweet roll, a bag of potato chips, lunch, a banana, a candy bar, a can of soda, a couple of cookies, dinner, a cookie, potato chips again, ice cream, a piece of fruit.

You need to record the eating event immediately because you can be unaware of much of your eating. The smog has hidden it from you. (See 2-H.) That's why diets fail, because everything is external.

After you have drawn your circles for a few days, you will see an eating pattern emerge. That's what Jackie, Linda, and Chris did. At first, I didn't want them to dwell on what they had eaten or why they had eaten it. I only wanted them to see the circles. Even though the eating pattern differed somewhat from day to day, over a period of a week they could see a distinctive pattern.

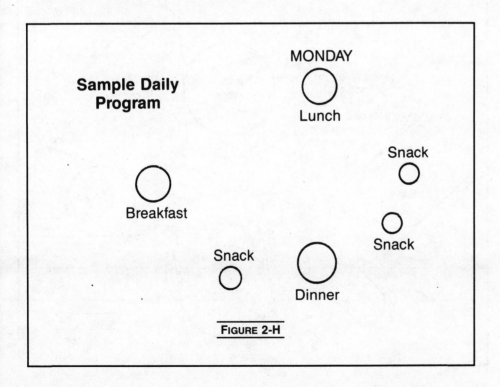

Sample Daily Program

MONDAY
Lunch

Snack

Breakfast

Snack

Snack

Dinner

FIGURE 2-H

Some people block out part of the pattern, not really wanting to admit to themselves how much and how often they eat.

Identifying an eating pattern sounds easy, doesn't it? And it is, even though some people block out part of the pattern, not really wanting to admit to themselves how much and how often they eat. Others don't count snacks or "just one bite" of something.

Every bite and snack is a legitimate eating event that calls for a circle. A circle begins when food of any kind goes into your mouth, and it ends when you stop eating. One handful of popcorn. Half a banana. A cup of coffee with cream and/or sugar.

Here is a tool to help you acknowledge that eating is happening and take charge of it. When you put food in your mouth, say aloud or think to yourself, "Start!" When you stop, say, "Stop!" Using those two words will affirm that you are eating and will strengthen you by demonstrating that you can and do stop eating. (See 2-I.)

People with weight problems are inclined to think that they are weak. They label themselves as bad because they can't stop eating. Often they're convinced that once they taste something good, they will never be able to stop eating.

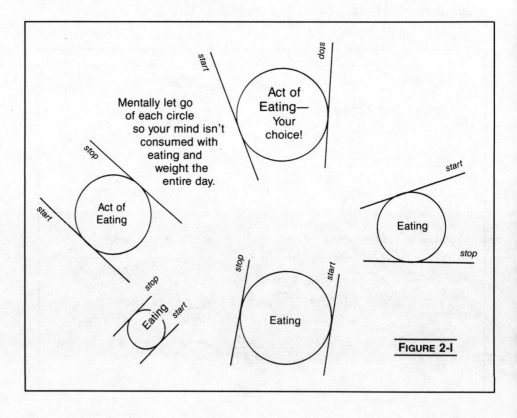

FIGURE 2-I

When clients say to me, "I can't eat just small amounts," I ask if at any time during the day they ate a small amount. After they think about it, they will recall a snack occasion. I point out that they're not weak because they were able to stop.

"But I'm bad. I couldn't stop until I had eaten three candy bars!"

"But you stopped after three," I point out.

Your mind will make the decision to stop when your body feels comfortable, before it feels stuffed. Your mind and body will work together consciously. So, each time you stop after you have eaten the amount you want, affirm yourself and remember that you did stop.

By using the words *start* and *stop* to reinforce the ability you have already, you will eventually recognize how you feel when you eat more than you want. Then you will be able to choose, as you did in this situation, to stop.

Anytime you make your circles, be kind to yourself. Don't get the self-criticism chatter going inside your head by putting value judgments on food. Food is food: it is not good or bad or fattening or forbidden. Food, in and of itself, is neutral; it is how you use it that can make the difference.

With food you live; without food you die. That makes it necessary. Isn't it lovely that you are also allowed to enjoy food? If food is essential and enjoyable, shouldn't it be something you *choose?*

By drawing the eating circles, you are creating a picture of your eating pattern which has been largely unconscious and uncontrolled. When you recognize the pattern as yours, you take possession of it. Then, and not until then, are you in a psychological position to discover its roots and change it if you choose. The boundaries you set for your eating should be carefully considered.

Work with the circles every day. To accept your eating pattern is to see that underneath the pattern lie clues—which we will unmask later—to why you eat as you do and what you can do to change the pattern if you choose. Thus, the circles will empower you to decide if you want to eat, how much, and when.

Before you begin using the circles—unless you have already begun, in which case, hooray for you!—I'd like you to think about three things.

1. All eating is by choice. You make a decision at some conscious or unconscious level about the food that does or does not go into your body. For example, if you eat four cookies, you chose to eat four. One cookie might have been enough. You could have eaten ten. You could

Your mind will make the decision to stop when your body feels comfortable, before it feels stuffed.

Food is food: it is not good or bad or fattening or forbidden.

The circles will empower you to decide if you want to eat, how much, and when.

have eaten a piece of pie or a banana, but you chose to eat four cookies.

If you go to bed tonight with a bloated stomach, you can choose your response.

2. *You don't have to fear failure* because Inner Eating is based not on achievement but on learning. You will learn, I promise you that; you have already learned by reading this far. You have discovered, for example, that if you go to bed tonight with a bloated stomach, you can choose your response.

You can feel guilty.

You can be angry with yourself.

Or you can say, "Well, I've learned something."

I urge you to choose the last one.

You'll start being aware of your discomfort at a conscious level.

Because you consider how you feel when you eat, you'll start being aware of your discomfort at a conscious level. You'll be aware *consciously* that you don't like that swollen, vaguely nauseated feeling. You'll want to change what made you feel that way, and you'll have the tools to do it.

3. *As you live with Inner Eating concepts, you'll remain the same person.* Inner Eating is a process incompatible with the idea that you are a thin person living inside an overstuffed body who wants to get out. This isn't a fat-thin issue. This is an issue of

> learning
>> your
>>> individual
>>>> internal
>>>>> boundaries.

NOTE TO MYSELF

I choose what and when I eat. I am responsible to myself for my food choices.

CHAPTER SUMMARY

Circles make visible your eating pattern and are a tool to aid conscious boundary building. Boundaries set limits and help define self. Healthy boundaries are firm but flexible. Diets offer people with weak boundaries a safety from fear of lack of control. Lack of boundaries acts like an internal smog to prevent clear thinking. Using circles to reveal eating patterns is equally useful for small and large weight problems. Circles encourage honesty with yourself and free you from preoccupation with food. Eating once a day sabotages the metabolism and may be the cause of your overweight. Every bite and nibble is a legitimate eating event. Using the words *start* and *stop* helps define eating occasions and demonstrates that you can and do stop eating.

STEPS TO BUILD ON

1. Every day draw on a piece of paper or in a notebook a circle to isolate and make visible each eating occasion.

2. To help you acknowledge each eating occasion, when you put the first piece of food into your mouth, say, "Start!" When you put the last piece in, say, "Stop!"

3. Notice the size of your circles, when you eat, and the pattern of eating your circles show. That is, do you eat a little all day or all at once? Or are there clusters of circles?

4. Don't scold yourself for your particular pattern of eating. There are no rights or wrongs, only learning about your eating pattern and its meaning and then deciding if you want to change any part of it.

5. Maintain your journal to cheer yourself on and to record your thoughts and feelings in this process.

NOTE

1. Bryant A. Stamford and Porter Shimer, *Fitness Without Exercise* (New York: Warner Books, 1990), p. 44.

3

Metabolism

"If I structured my life so that I had just my regular meals," Frema-jane said, "I'm sure I'd be okay. I have this terrible habit of eating between meals."

"Do you like to eat three regular meals?" I asked. "Every day?"

"Sometimes," she said, "but not always."

"Isn't it okay *not* to eat just three daily meals?"

The shock on her face made me realize how radical my words sounded. "Shouldn't I be eating just meals with nothing in between?"

"I don't," I said.

Her eyes widened in shock a second time. "You don't?"

"Why be so rigid?" I asked. "After all, there's no right and wrong about this. Be creative. Find out what works best for you."

Find out what works best for you.

Fremajane, a battered veteran of many diets and an erratic pattern of childhood eating, could hardly believe what I said. For her, three meals represented perfect eating, something she was always striving for and never seeming to achieve. Frequently she nibbled between meals—and always felt guilty because she nibbled.

What is a meal? *Meal* is a word that creates an image in people's minds. Perhaps they carry memories from childhood of large family dinners. That image, or definition of a meal, gets in the way of their ability to see meals also as small eating occasions. Then when they try to eat small amounts, they are apt to avoid "meals" because they don't want to eat large amounts. Whether it's called a meal or a snack, it's a legitimate eating occasion.

┌─ NOTE TO MYSELF ─────────────────────┐
│ *All eating occasions count, whether they're called* │
│ *snacks, nibbles, or meals.* │
└──────────────────────────────────────┘

Are you locked into eating exactly three meals?

What about the number of times you eat each day? Are you locked into eating exactly three meals? What happens if you eat breakfast and feel starved by ten o'clock? Can you eat something without guilt? Or lunchtime comes and you think, *I'm not very hungry.* What do you do then?

Metabolism refers to the rate at which your body converts food into energy (which it burns) or fat (which it stores).

You don't have to despair or feel guilty about varying from your normal eating pattern. If hunger strikes you at other than the "normal times," your body is speaking to you. Listen to it. Likely your body has burned all its fuel and is telling you that it's ready for more food. Metabolism, or your metabolic rate, refers to the rate at which your body converts food into energy (which it burns) or fat (which it stores).

In this chapter we'll talk about number of meals per day. As a way to lose weight, some people resort to one-meal-a-day dieting. This method is fairly common among men. It works like this: because you ate heavily at night, the next morning you may not be very hungry. So you don't eat all day. Then at night when your metabolism naturally slows down, you eat a big dinner.

One meal is the least effective way to cope with weight problems.

The once-daily plan gets you fighting against the natural working process of your body. Along with the top researchers, I'm convinced that one meal is the *least effective* way to cope with weight problems.

I have three objections to this method.

1. The once-a-day pattern tends to turn into gorging. You finally eat at the end of the day and intend to stop at a certain point. But after you've denied yourself food all day, you find you don't want to stop.

It normally takes five or six hours to process an entire meal into an energy-producing or a fat-producing form.

2. Because you limited your food to one meal, during the rest of the day your body behaved as if it were being starved. Actually, you *were* starving your body because it normally takes five or six hours to process an entire meal into an energy-producing or a fat-producing

form. When you hold back the food, the body slows down the metabolism, and the body preserves its energy.

3. Whenever you eat a large amount of food at one time, your body can't accommodate it. Being the efficient machine it is, your body stores the excess. If you overeat repeatedly, your body becomes remarkably efficient at converting your food into fat and storing it. Result: weight gain.

Your body becomes remarkably efficient at converting your food into fat and storing it.

Studies in nutrition suggest that many people do better eating several meals a day. One word being used for this is *grazing*. Advocates point out that many animals don't eat one large meal, but they graze, eating a little now and a little more later. Throughout the day they feed on the grass around them. Nibblers or grazers tend to handle weight better because their bodies don't get glutted with food and store much of it as fat.

Nibblers or grazers tend to handle weight better because their bodies don't get glutted with food and store much of it as fat.

Please understand, *grazing implies that the day's total food intake won't be greater than a normal day's eating.* It does *not* suggest continual stuffing.

Dr. Bryant Stamford, head of the Health Promotion and Wellness Center at the University of Louisville, says the center's current research shows that the worst possible way to eat and to care for the body is to have one massive meal a day, which is fairly common. He says the second worst way is to eat only two meals a day or no breakfast, a large lunch, and a larger dinner.

The research at the center points now to the fact that if individuals don't *increase* their total amount of food but stretch it over several meals a day, they store less fat.

If individuals don't increase their total amount of food but stretch it over several meals a day, they store less fat.

Research shows that many people who are obese eat less than people of normal weight but make the mistake . . . of skipping meals to be able to eat one big one. In one study, fully 80 percent of the obese people surveyed were eating less than people of normal weight but were making the "one big meal a day" mistake. Big meals tends to produce big waistlines.[1]

Bryant Stamford's research indicates strongly that adults who spread their *total intake* into smaller meals throughout the day will be leaner than those who eat larger but fewer meals.

Adults who spread their total intake into smaller meals throughout the day will be leaner than those who eat larger but fewer meals.

The studies at the University of Louisville and other places involve counting calories—which I don't advocate. Even so, calorie counting makes the plan more readily understandable.

It works like this. Suppose you decide that you will eat 1,800 calories a day. You can eat your total calories in any number of ways.

You could do some simple dividing. You could eat 600 calories three times a day. Or you might decide to have 300 calories for breakfast, 800 for lunch, and the final 700 for dinner.

As we've discussed, the worst decision would be to go without food all day and then eat all 1,800 calories at one time in the evening. Because your body can burn only so many calories at a time, a large part of your 1,800 would be held over and stored as fat.

However, if you decide on a total consumption of 1,800 calories and you spread it over five or six meals a day, your body would easily burn all the calories between feedings. Using this method, according to Stamford, you could eat 1,800 calories and not create any fat as residue. (See 3-A.)

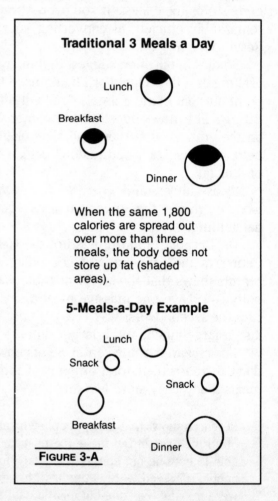

Traditional 3 Meals a Day

Lunch

Breakfast

Dinner

When the same 1,800 calories are spread out over more than three meals, the body does not store up fat (shaded areas).

5-Meals-a-Day Example

Lunch

Snack

Snack

Breakfast

Dinner

FIGURE 3-A

If you decide to try six meals a day (or any other variation), remember to count your circle of containment—a beginning and an ending—each time and resolve that you are going to enjoy eating your food. By following these simple reminders, you'll probably eat less food each day. With a five- or six-meals-a-day plan, you're never stuffed at any meal, and you're never uncomfortably hungry throughout the day.

Our society actually accommodates itself nicely to this type of spaced eating. Many offices and businesses allow a ten- to fifteen-minute coffee break in the morning and again in the afternoon. If you're a student, you usually have five or ten minutes between classes. Others, who time isn't so structured, can easily choose when they want to eat.

If this idea seems revolutionary, you might talk with someone who has traveled in England. A friend I'll call Bob had this experience. "You know what amazed me the most?" he said. "Their eating habits."

He noticed that few English people were overweight. He then explained about their meals. "Before breakfast, they had a cup of tea, nothing else, although they used milk and sugar. Breakfast followed an hour later. In the middle of the morning they had morning tea or coffee that included sandwiches. No matter where we were or what we were doing, everything stopped for tea. Lunch came two or three hours after tea. They had another tea around four o'clock with food, and then an evening meal—fairly light—about 8:00 P.M. Six times every day. And that was it."

Bob was amazed at first because he thought that they should all be twice their weight. Then he observed that although they had plenty of food around them, including a lot of sweet things, they didn't eat much at any one time. "I'd never heard of such an idea," he said, as one who came from rigid three-meals-a-day home.

However, because most Americans grew up eating three meals a day, they have difficulty trying anything different. Why not rethink your eating pattern? Choose for yourself.

When the clock dictates your normal meal times, ask yourself,

- Am I really hungry?
- Am I eating from habit?
- Am I eating now because that's what everybody else does?
- Am I snacking/grazing, thinking I won't have to count this as eating? (All eating counts!)

If you discover that eating more than three meals a day works for you, do it.

For many, frequent meals throughout the day work. But there are three things to remember.

With a five- or six-meals-a-day plan, you're never stuffed at any meal, and you're never uncomfortably hungry throughout the day.

Although they had plenty of food around them . . . they didn't eat much at any one time.

Why not rethink your eating pattern?

1. Don't starve yourself.
2. Eat more often *if you choose.*
3. Listen to your body's hunger signals.

┌─ **NOTE TO MYSELF** ──────────────────┐

*Several small meals ease my desire to eat
large amounts.*

└─────────────────────────────────────┘

─────────────── □ ───────────────

When I first suggested eating more often, one woman panicked. "I just barely control myself now with only three meals a day. Then sometimes I end up gorging anyway. If I decided to eat four or six times a day . . ."

"That's the point," I said. "You might not feel the need to gorge yourself if you know that you can eat again in two hours."

"That never occurred to me," she said. She tried eating less food and more often. After a few weeks she realized that the method worked well for her.

Problems involving fear tend to crop up when I suggest eating more than three daily meals. Many are afraid of the freedom, because freedom means possibly going totally out of control. They fear they'll start to nibble and not be able to stop.

"It takes practice," I tell them, "but keep working at it. You can do it."

┌─ **NOTE TO MYSELF** ──────────────────┐

*Each time I eat, I know I can eat again when I
get hungry.*

└─────────────────────────────────────┘

Judy was raised to eat three meals a day, all of them large. She cheated—as she called it—by eating more times during the day.

"If you're hungry, Judy, listen to the hunger. Accept it," I said. "Keep monitoring yourself. You don't have to eat until you're very full; you can teach yourself when to stop."

Her problem was physiological. Judy's metabolism couldn't handle three big meals with nothing in between. After a large meal she would feel sluggish. Because of the hours between meals, as she got hungry, she also felt physically weak, but it wasn't time to eat so she couldn't do anything except "cheat." Judy realized that she couldn't live comfortably on only three meals. Her metabolism required six small meals a day.

---NOTE TO MYSELF---

Small, frequent meals may feel good in my head and in my stomach.

Since large meals trigger extra amounts of insulin to break down the food, they also promote the conversion of carbohydrates, which include sugar, into fat. By spreading her total food intake over several circles, Judy's daily activities burned them up. She began losing her weight. For her, it was a matter of learning to cooperate with her body instead of working against it. Slowly Judy learned to listen to her body's signals, and she arrived at a sensible eating pattern for her.

Understanding the role of metabolism in eating will help you decide on your number of circles and how much food each circle will hold. If you're like most people, your blood sugar level drops around four o'clock in the afternoon. You become sluggish, perhaps irritable. Some people get woozy, can't think, and even tremble. You need food to satisfy your body's needs—which is one signal you learn to note. Why not have a small snack then? Decide on an apple, half a sandwich, whatever you're hungry for—enough to raise your blood sugar level, yet not enough to make a full meal. This amount then carries you over until dinner.

Audrey DeLaMartre learned to understand and appreciate my process. She said as she cut down on food intake and experimented with the content and placement of her food-occasion circles, she learned that three meals plus an afternoon snack per day kept her in a comfort zone between slightly hungry and slightly full.

"Because of my work, I have to sit a lot, and snacking is easy and a real temptation between 10:30 A.M. and 4:00 P.M. I was delighted to

Since large meals trigger extra amounts of insulin to break down the food, they also promote the conversion of carbohydrates, which include sugar, into fat.

discover that if I ate a low-calorie *hot* lunch—I really enjoy Lean Cuisine—at 11:00 A.M. or 11:30 A.M., and one scoop of frozen fruit yogurt at 3:00 P.M., I could reduce my unnecessary extra snacking. My energy was high and I felt good, I wanted less supper, and the pounds I had gained from sitting began to melt away. A hot lunch was a significant discovery."

The purpose of food is to keep your energy level up throughout the day.

When you learn to listen to your body and practice doing it, you'll achieve the normal eating pattern for *you*. Because each of us is different, you can't judge the right amount by observing anyone else. The purpose of food is to keep your energy level up throughout the day. And only you, working with your body, can make that decision.

Some days you may need more food than others, or you may want to eat less than on other days.

Your body will ask for what it needs, sometimes in the form of a craving. However, your unique body may not give you the same messages every day. Some days you may need more food than others, or different kinds of foods, or you may want to eat less than on other days. Dr. Larry Covin, who has no weight problem, told me that at times he'll eat only once a day because that's what he wants. He eats when he's hungry, sometimes he doesn't; he isn't hung up on the issue. Which comes to my main point on the subject. Newer research challenges these ideas about metabolism. Because research is always in the process of uncovering knowledge, what is an absolute one day may turn out later to be just the opposite. So as you read and learn about your body, remember also to trust your own instincts.

Eat what's right for you.

Take breakfast. Since infancy you have probably heard that everybody needs to start the day with a good breakfast. Some say that concept began as a sales gimmick by makers of breakfast cereal, an idea they continued to stress, and eventually it came to be accepted without question by most people. That may be true.

But some people just aren't hungry in the morning. If you're not hungry, don't eat; wait until you are hungry. This is the difference between skipping a meal to lose weight versus not eating because you're not hungry.

No matter how many daily meals you decide on, approach each meal by saying,

"I am now starting a new circle, and it will end when I finish eating."

"I am creating boundaries to my eating."

"I will choose the number of times I eat by how hungry I am."

When you do eat, enjoy your food in the environment that you choose. If you like a pleasant setting when you eat, create that atmosphere. If you like well-presented food, respond to that. For some people, neither is important. You may be just as comfortable eating while standing in the kitchen. If so, that's what you do. Whatever your style, know when you begin eating and when you end.

If you like a pleasant setting when you eat, create that atmosphere.

Allow yourself the freedom not to enjoy a meal. For example, at breakfast you may prefer eating a dull cereal that you know will hold you until your next meal while enjoying the mental stimulation of the morning newspaper. That's okay. It's your choice.

In addition, if your time is short and allows only for a takeout from the deli, it may not be a feast, but it will hold you until dinner. Quick food is a valid choice that you may or may not enjoy. Just be aware of when you start and stop, and if your body needs it.

Quick food is a valid choice that you may or may not enjoy.

NOTE TO MYSELF

I'm free not to enjoy every meal.

As you begin to listen to your body, you'll discover your balance point—the comfortable zone between feeling hungry and stuffed.

NOTE TO MYSELF

Today I ate too much. I won't beat myself up about it, but I will remember how it feels.

CHAPTER SUMMARY

Having three meals a day is not the only valid eating model. Six small meals may be more comfortable and reduce total food consumption. A meal is any eating occasion. Eating one meal a day in the evening is the hardest for the body to metabolize, so it stores the food as fat. A craving is a body's way of calling for what it needs. Grazing is a legitimate form of eating small meals and getting a low-calorie intake. Stop eating when you're no longer hungry. How fast your metabolism burns the food determines how often you require food. The purpose of food is to maintain your energy level. Eat in the atmosphere you prefer. Feel free not to focus on your food when you eat.

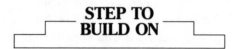

STEP TO BUILD ON

1. Experiment with spreading your total food intake over several meals each day to find a structure that serves your best comfort and energy level.

NOTE

1. Bryant A. Stamford and Porter Shimer, *Fitness Without Exercise* (New York: Warner Books, 1990), p. 128.

4

The Nutrition Quandary

Cathy, like many of us, has been bombarded with so much nutritional information that she no longer can choose the food she wants to eat. She no longer knows. (See 4-A.)

Eating only for nutrition denies that we want, even need, other things that taste good. We have interpreted this nutrition information to mean that we *can't* eat, for example, a candy bar. Both taste and nutrition are important, and they are not mutually exclusive.

You don't need to be a nutrition expert to make informed choices. When helping people make choices, I stress that food is food; no food is inherently bad or good. No food is totally lacking in nutritional value, although some are more nutrient-packed than others. As I stress throughout this book, *variety* is the first ingredient of sound nutrition.

Variety is the first ingredient of sound nutrition.

For at least the past fifty years, nutritionists have urged us to eat daily from each of the four food groups, or sometimes called the basic four. The "basic four" are milk, meat, fruit and vegetable, and grain (bread and cereal).

The "basic four" are milk, meat, fruit and vegetable, and grain (bread and cereal).

Covert Bailey lectures extensively on nutrition, physical fitness, and body fat. He heads the Bailey Fit-or-Fat Center and has several advanced degrees, most notably a master of science in nutritional biochemistry from the Massachusetts Institute of Technology. I'm indebted to Bailey, who recommends a balanced diet and then gives three rules of selecting foods that are

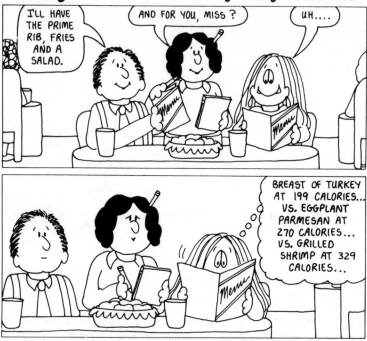

FIGURE 4-A

1. low in fat.
2. low in sugar.
3. high in fiber.

Like Bailey, I urge my clients to eat a balanced diet—often the most neglected aspect of diet books.

But what is a balanced diet?

Here is a circle showing the four food groups. (See 4-B.)

According to Covert Bailey, the easiest way for most adults to get a balanced diet with all the necessary protein, vitamins, and minerals is to eat two meats, two milks, four breads/cereals, and four fruits/vegetables.[1] This is bare-bones nutrition and as much information as most people need without getting bogged down like poor Cathy.

If you want to pursue the subject, I offer these suggestions to provide nutrition and variety in your daily food intake.

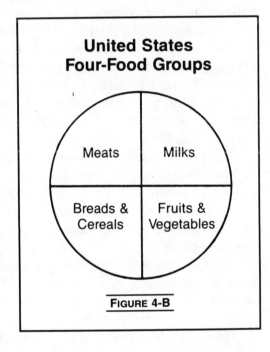

United States Four-Food Groups

Meats | Milks

Breads & Cereals | Fruits & Vegetables

FIGURE 4-B

1. Use the guidelines of the federal government's Recommended Daily Allowances (RDA), the American Heart Association, or the National Cancer Institute, but don't turn them into rigid eating rules.

Don't turn guidelines into rigid eating rules.

2. Consider your sense of taste. For instance, if you don't like fish, don't eat it. Choose chicken or turkey.

3. Eat the energy-producing nutrients, but limit your intake of fat. (Fat is a *stored* fuel source.)

Fat is a stored fuel source.

In *The California Nutrition Book* the authors say:

You should be aware that even average men and women are decidedly unaverage in a good many ways. Each of us has a unique set of nutritional needs, the result of heredity, lifestyle, foodstyle, age, sex, the demands we make on our bodies, and the demands we do not make on them.[2]

———————————— □ ————————————

Several of my clients have come to me for assistance at a time when nutritional information had become more important than choice, to the point that they could hardly choose anymore. They feared that if they ate outside the guidelines, they would lose control.

For example, one woman with whom I worked was very self-controlled and self-restricting, and she feared making choices. Occasionally she and her husband went from Minneapolis to New York for business meetings. Before they left, she telephoned the restaurant where they would eat to find out if the food listed on her current diet was available there.

Most people aren't that self-restricted, but many have trouble making choices and depend on packaged diet meals to control their weight. An example is Dr. Scott Northey. To add to his dilemma, his wife is an excellent cook. She and their two daughters have learned to listen to their bodies and have developed a strong sense of internal boundaries.

One evening, Scott took out his premeasured food in its plastic container and started to mix the powdered eggs. His daughters silently watched him prepare his packaged food.

"Yuck!" said one of them.

"How can you eat that stuff?" asked the other.

They were enjoying delicious food, and he had only powdered eggs.

Scott looked down at his powdered, prepared meal and then over at the food on the table. They were enjoying delicious food, and he had only powdered eggs. He laughed, too.

Scott realized he had given up his freedom to choose food for himself. He is now grappling with gaining control of his choices.

Dr. Henry Cloud says of choices:

We need to be aware of and own . . . our choices. . . . *Choices are not true choices unless we are aware of all the feelings, attitudes, behaviors, wants, thoughts, and abilities that go into them.* To own and make our choices, we must be aware of all the aspects of ourselves that go into any decision. In addition, we must be aware that we are making a choice about almost everything we do. There is no stronger element to forging an identity than owning and taking responsibility for choices. It is the cornerstone of freedom, love, and responsibility.[3]

NOTE TO MYSELF

Learning to make choices about food will strengthen my ability to make choices in other areas of my life.

There is Hillary, who is Jewish. She had a similar fear of choices when she attended functions such as an Oneg Shabbat. She would stare at the long tables filled with sweets. "I have this terrible fear that if I start to eat one dessert, I'll clean out the place," she said.

"You can learn to go to any kind of party or celebration and make choices," I told her.

"With all that food staring back at me?" she asked as if she thought I was crazy. "You don't know how weak I am."

"Think about this," I said. "The next time you go to such a celebration, look over everything available. Then decide on the very best treat—the one you would like to eat more than anything else on the table. If you can't decide on just one, narrow your choice to two. Then put the dessert or desserts you choose on your plate. Before you take your first bite, say to yourself, 'I'm going to enjoy eating this.'"

"The next time you go to such a celebration, look over everything available. Then decide on the very best treat."

"Then what?"

"Eat the food one bite at a time. Eat slowly and enjoy every bite. When you feel your enjoyment beginning to leave—when you've had enough—just stop. Quit! If necessary, put down your plate and walk away."

A short time later, Hillary did exactly that. At a social event she walked the full length of the table and paused to ask herself, Which one do I really want to eat? "You know, just then I felt as if food wasn't in charge of my life," she said. "I was making the decision."

Unable to settle on one, Hillary selected two desserts and then sat down at a table to eat. Just before she took the first bite, she said softly to herself, "I'm going to enjoy this."

She said softly to herself, "I'm going to enjoy this."

"Tell me, Hillary," I said, already suspecting I knew part of the answer, "how much did you actually eat?"

"It's hard for me to believe that I actually made my own choices."

"That's what's so amazing. With the first dessert, I finished maybe a third of it. And with the other, less than a quarter." She was bursting with joy as she added, "I felt I was in control instead of the food controlling me. It's hard for me to believe that I actually made my own choices. I limited how much I wanted, and everything was coming from my decisions." Hillary has remained at her desired weight for over five years.

Here's another example. Rollie and I chatted at a tennis party. "I've heard about your upcoming book," he said. "I've always had trouble with my weight. What's your philosophy?"

Because we had only a few minutes, I explained the basics to him quickly.

Rollie then told me that he remembered one time at breakfast when he stopped eating at the balance point—the point that he was comfortable. "I decided that when I had enough, I'd get up from the table." And that's exactly what he did.

He said, "You know, if I could eat like that all the time, I wouldn't have a weight problem."

"You *can* eat like that all the time!" I told him.

┌─ **NOTE TO MYSELF** ──────────────────┐

I can choose what I want to eat.

└──┘

Choice is difficult for most people to grasp.

Choice is difficult for most people to grasp. Because they haven't learned balance, which is what I emphasize, they tend toward one of two extremes. Either they satisfy their taste buds by eating whatever appeals to them and overeat, or they decide to eat nutritiously and deny their taste buds.

If they're hungry and pay attention only to taste, they may eat only candy bars. Today we have enough variety in candy bars that they could go for days with nothing else. But eventually their bodies would rebel and crave something more nutritious. They need to combine their taste choices with their knowledge of nutrition, which includes low-fat, low-sugar and complex carbohydrate foods. It's not simply one or the other.

A significant study done by Barbara Rolls of Johns Hopkins University states that the human body craves variety. The more you eat of a specific food, the less its appeal. When you rigidly follow a restrictive diet, you don't have enough variety in your food. No matter how nutritional a diet is, Dr. Rolls says that it can work against you because you're setting yourself up to fail. It's normal and natural for your body to start craving the "forbidden foods."

In an article about Dr. Rolls's research, Ellen Shell writes,

> Any strict diet is an attempt to override the body's natural hungers— including others, the hunger for variety. . . . The very process of dieting may bring on abnormal behavior patterns.[4]

The human body craves variety. The more you eat of a specific food, the less its appeal.

For example, Phyllis is beautiful, athletic, and slender. When we talked, she was thinking of entering a triathlon. Judging from her physical appearance alone, I would have considered her one of the last people in the world to have trouble making choices.

As we discussed choices, Phyllis laughed. "Minutes before we started to talk, I was thinking about eating. Inside my head I was saying, 'If I want to be really *good,* I'll just have fruit.' If I give in to what I'd like, I'd have cookies and flavored yogurt. Then I'd feel guilty for eating those things. I didn't consider that there might be a way to get my tastes satisfied and still eat nutritionally."

"If I give in to what I'd like, I'd have cookies and flavored yogurt. Then I'd feel guilty for eating those things."

Phyllis and I were still talking about her choice of fruit or cookies and yogurt when her boyfriend walked up. Like Phyllis, he's tall, slender, and athletic looking. Just then Phyllis said, "You know I might just have a cookie."

"But you might get fat if you do," he said.

Without his being aware of the impact of his words, he was doing what countless others do—categorizing foods as thin or fat. Among other things, categorizing eliminates choices.

Among other things, categorizing eliminates choices.

If you're a veteran of diet programs, you know how this goes. You get caught in the labeling trap, and after a while your body craves variety beyond what it's getting, so you break away from the diet. But because you don't know how to take charge of "bad" food, you binge. Then a terrible feeling of guilt follows.

If you label some food as bad, you begin to say things like,

"I can't eat sugar. Sugar is bad."

"Food with a high-fat content is bad."

"Chocolate is bad because it makes me fat."

It's not the food that's bad; it's the *amount* that creates problems. Deleting these foods from your food list doesn't eliminate them from your diet anyway. In fact, designating them as forbidden may make them more appealing.

The biggest problems come from restrictions of any kind. Carrots, for example, are good for us. But if we ate only carrots, they would become a poor source of nutrition, not bad food. Or eating just potatoes. Or only milk. No food is bad; only how we choose to use it can make it less than healthful for us. Food is neutral, blameless.

No food is bad; only how we choose to use it can make it less than healthful for us. Food is neutral, blameless.

Even more unreasonable, labeling food good or bad encourages us to lift the label off the food and paste it on ourselves, and we become good or bad for our use of it. Therefore, when you want to be bad, you eat food you've labeled bad. If you want to punish yourself, you opt for the food you consider inferior, like "junk" food. If you restrict yourself, you may grow tired of the rules and restrictions, eat "bad" food, and end up with a heavy load of guilt. I want to help you eliminate blame and guilty feelings from food and eating.

Don't use food as a reason to beat up on yourself. You're not bad, either.

It's equally important for you to realize that you must not transfer the good-bad labels to yourself. Don't use food as a reason to beat up on yourself. You're not bad, either. If you've had problems with food, you've probably learned some negative concepts. But you're in the process of changing that.

Despite what I say, some people persist with questions like, "Isn't food with a high-fat content bad?" Again, it's not the food itself that's bad, but the amount you eat and the variety. *Nutritionally,* you may choose to limit your fat intake, but it's a decision you make for yourself.

Fats are not bad, according to Paul Saltman, Joel Gurin, and Ira Mothner in *The California Nutrition Book*.

Fats play a major role in making eating one of life's more rewarding experiences. Take the fats out of food and you strip away much of its taste and flavor as well as its fat-soluble vitamins. Think of the smell of roasting meat or frying onions, the way ice cream glides along your tongue, the crunch of corn and potato chips, the tangy taste of sharp cheeses, or what butter and sour cream do for baked potatoes.

"Fats have what nutritionists call satiety value."

Even if you have little taste for fat, your stomach is still likely to find it the most satisfying of foodstuffs. Fats have what nutritionists call satiety value. Meals that contain a good deal of fat remain in the stomach much longer than meals that do not. So you are likely to stay satisfied quite a bit longer if you dine on fried chicken and buttered biscuits than on chef's salad and melba toast.[5]

However, if you eat large amounts of food high in fat, you're not being considerate of your body. If you stay in tune with your body and how it feels after you overeat high-fat food, you'll notice that you soon begin to feel sluggish. High energy is what you want, not sluggishness, and listening to your body is the key to balancing your intake of foods to achieve a maximum energy level.

Consider the examples of Cindy and Linda.

Cindy decided that she weighed too much. To conquer this problem, she studied nutrition, particularly fat grams. She became so knowledgeable about fat grams that she could tell which brand of skim milk had fewer fat grams than another. However, at times she found herself eating food high in fat, and she felt guilty. She didn't know to control the amounts. As a result she would overeat high-fat foods, and although she felt guilty, she didn't want to own her excessive eating of them. Eventually she developed bulimia.

She became so knowledgeable about fat grams that she could tell which brand of skim milk had fewer fat grams than another.

Linda told me about eating French fries and a hamburger, quite aware that overeating these items causes extra weight. Instead of saying, "Linda, you can't have such food if you want to lose weight!" I asked, "How did you feel after you had eaten the fries and hamburger?"

"Sluggish," she said, "and heavy."

"Do you like that feeling?"

"No, of course not," she said.

"Then that's the reason you may want to avoid overeating them. Not because you *can't* have them, but because you don't want that sluggish feeling they cause. You'd like to feel energized by your food. If you discover that even small amounts make you feel sluggish, you can decide which is more important—how the food tastes or how your body feels."

"If you discover that even small amounts make you feel sluggish, you can decide which is more important— how the food tastes or how your body feels."

Linda thought about her answers to my questions and cut down on her fat intake by listening to her body and understanding nutrition. She did not follow Cindy's example. When Cindy concentrated only on the number of fat grams, she wasn't listening to her body. She was making her decision from external factors, not her own very personal and valid physical evidence.

When I talk to clients about food, I keep returning to one important point—how the body feels. I ask frequently, "After you ate that, how did your body feel?"

If you make your choices based on how your body feels, you can choose not to eat a specific food again or to eat it rarely. Instead of fighting your taste buds, work with your body, including your sense of taste, by focusing on how it feels.

Work with your body, including your sense of taste.

You can learn to listen to your body by asking yourself,

- What does this taste like?
- What does it feel like in my mouth?
- How do I feel after I've eaten it?
- Is my body telling me that I've had enough?

For example, chocolate gets labeled a bad food. When clients start telling me about all their problems with chocolate, I ask, "Do you like chocolate? Really like chocolate?"

"Oh, yes," they always answer.

"Satisfy your taste buds with quality instead of quantity."

"Then why not buy the best quality chocolates? Satisfy your taste buds with quality instead of quantity. You'll feel satisfied with less candy, and you can enjoy every bite because you're not sitting in judgment against yourself."

My friend Audrey found this the most helpful solution to what she had once referred to as her "addiction" to chocolate. By removing the labels of "bad" and "addiction" and focusing on her enjoyment of the chocolate rather than guilt, she ate less chocolate and enjoyed it more. Putting the "chocolate occasion" in a circle not only gave it a beginning and an ending, but it became a little party she created for herself that she didn't need to keep repeating. She had created her own boundaries.

The more foods you eliminate, the more you restrict your choices. Avoiding bad foods then becomes more powerful than eating from choice.

Labeling, judging, and categorizing foods usually mean eliminating them. The more foods you eliminate, the more you restrict your choices. *Avoiding bad foods* then becomes more powerful than eating from choice because you've never been taught that choice is the opposite of control.

┌─ **NOTE TO MYSELF** ─────────────────────────┐
│ *There are no bad foods, only nutritional differences.* │
└──┘

For people with eating problems, such an idea poses a frightening prospect. "If I had a kitchen filled with food, I'd be afraid that I'd go on an eating binge and never stop as long as one cracker remained," said one woman. Although she probably wouldn't eat that much, her fear is real and significant. Her fear is as strong as reality for her, and such a possibility is just too much for her to risk. Having a variety of food available to her is like dumping a person into the deepest part of the lake and saying, "Learn to swim."

If you are caught up in labeling and restricting your variety, an easy way out is to start with the basic concept of circles. Within those boundaries, your own boundaries, you slowly add some foods you've avoided because they tasted so good and you were afraid you couldn't stop eating.

Start with the foods you love, but learn to limit the amounts by your conscious decision. Tell yourself, "I'll eat two slices of bread" or "I'll eat one muffin." If you eat one too many this time, don't beat up on yourself. You'll do it next time because it will be easier. And it keeps getting easier.

Tell yourself, "I'll eat two slices of bread" or "I'll eat one muffin." If you eat one too many this time, don't beat up on yourself. You'll do it next time because it will be easier.

When chronic dieters label and subsequently eliminate specific foods, they lose their sense of being satisfied and enjoying their food. For Hillary, she loved bread but felt she should eliminate it if she was trying to lose weight. As a result, she ended up bingeing on bread and felt guilty. Bread became the bad food—and when she overate on it, she was "bad."

"Try this instead," I said. "Eat the same meal as your family." (Hillary usually ate a diet meal and watched her family enjoy their food. Later she would binge on bread.) "Include bread as part of your meal. Remind yourself that bread is on the table if you want to eat it, but you don't have to eat it."

"Eat the same meal as your family."

Initially, the idea scared her, but she decided to try. At first she ate a lot of bread, but over a period of weeks her intense desire for great amounts of it eased. "I figured out that I didn't feel deprived of my favorite food."

At first she ate a lot of bread, but over a period of weeks her intense desire for great amounts of it eased.

In time she balanced her meals and found them satisfying emotionally, physically, and nutritionally. By then she had developed a healthier relationship with food, she enjoyed it more, and she started to lose weight.

———————————— □ ————————————

Here are four simple guidelines about choice in the Inner Eating process.

1. Cut out the foods you don't like.
2. Eliminate the times you don't need food.
3. Don't eliminate foods you enjoy.
4. Learn to limit the amounts of the foods you enjoy.

———————————— □ ————————————

Hillary loved ice cream, but it was on her bad-food list.

Hillary, also, loved ice cream, but it was on her bad-food list. Once while she was shopping for groceries, the store was offering sample cones of a new brand of ice cream. Rather than accept a free cone and allow it to be a circle of containment, she had an inner dialogue that went something like this: *I can't eat ice cream if I want to lose weight. But my husband can eat ice cream. I know what I'll do. I'll buy a half gallon of ice cream for him.*

Before she realized what she had done, Hillary had eaten half the carton of ice cream.

When Hillary got home, even before she had taken off her coat, she opened the ice-cream carton and used a large spoon to scoop out the slushy half-frozen part. "Just a taste," she told herself. You can probably guess the rest this story. Before she realized what she had done, Hillary had eaten half the carton of ice cream.

"Tell me, Hillary," I said, "if you had scooped all of that ice cream into a bowl, would you have eaten that much?"

"Why, no, of course not!"

"If you had put the ice cream into a bowl, you might have limited the amount because you could see how much you were going to eat."

"You see, if you had put the ice cream in a bowl, it would have represented one defined circle. If you had put the ice cream into a bowl, you might have limited the amount because you could see how much you were going to eat. If you had put a small amount into a small bowl and eaten it slowly, you would have enjoyed the taste just as much, maybe more, and you would have had the added psychological pleasure of defining your boundaries. That's how you set your limits before you start to eat."

Because Hillary's thoughts had been about *not* eating, she had given no serious consideration to taking charge of her eating.

Chris loved brownies. She could eat a whole pan of them. She loved them more than any other food. To help herself get past her compulsion of eliminating brownies and eventually bingeing on them, she decided to finish off every meal with her formerly forbidden food. She would tell herself, "I am going to close this meal with one brownie. At the next meal, I can have another."

Christ had several things working for her. First, she chose a desirable food that previously she had labeled forbidden. Second, by eating a brownie at every meal—if she wanted it—she minimized her fear of overindulging in one item. Third, any food she ate every day, several times a day, would tend to lose its appeal to her. Also, she was doing away with the self-criticism and self-judgment for what she really wanted to eat. Finally, Chris was setting everything in motion so that she could ask herself what she would like to eat.

Do you see yourself in Hillary or Chris? It's easy to get caught the way they were if you label foods as

good.
    bad.
        junk.
            really nutritious.
            healthful.
            pleasurable.

Instead of trying to label them, evaluate them using the three guidelines of taste, nutritional content, and the effect on your body.

The effect on your body, or how you feel after eating a particular food, may have to do with the amount you consume. If you eat too much, you may feel lethargic because you're uncomfortable, not because you are reacting to the food. Other foods may make you feel sluggish or nauseated, no matter how little you eat. That's when you have to decide if the taste is worth the feeling you have afterward. You may decide you should avoid the food. Only you can make that choice. The way your body reacts is one key for making a choice. You will know how to choose if you listen to your body.

You will know how to choose if you listen to your body.

———————— □ ————————

To help people make choices, we list the foods they like especially well. Then we use a grid to sort out which foods they like most and which ones they only believe they prefer.[6]

The grid helps them make and prioritize choices and understand that they can make decisions about food.

I want people to see that the choices are their own, not mine, and not made to please anyone else. By placing decisions back in the hands of my clients and assuring them that they have the wisdom and strength to make the changes they feel are wisest, my program affirms and validates each individual. The grid helps them make and prioritize choices and understand that they can make decisions about food. They learn that

- they are helping themselves.
- they are being responsible for their eating.
- they are acknowledging their unique tastes.

How the Grid Works

Suppose that I ask Stephanie, "What foods do you enjoy eating? Name six of them."

Stephanie lists the following:

1. ice cream
2. strawberries
3. chocolate fudge
4. bagels
5. raspberries
6. shrimp

"You have selected six foods," I tell her. "Now I want you to compare them with each other. First, let's compare ice cream and strawberries. Which do you like better?"

"Strawberries," Stephanie answers.

This is the first comparison, and I circle 2. Next I ask her to compare ice cream with chocolate fudge. She chooses the fudge, and I circle 3. Then she compares ice cream with bagels. Stephanie does this until she has gone through all six foods.

That completed, she goes through the list again, comparing strawberries with fudge, then with bagels. She continues to compare until she has indicated her preference for each item in her cluster with every other item.

When she finishes, the grid looks like this. (See 4-C.)

Stephanie is amazed that she put raspberries and strawberries above chocolate fudge. (Clients often surprise themselves like this.) Until now she might have said she was addicted to chocolate, especially to chocolate fudge. (Frankly, I think that the word *addiction* is used far too casually.) But Stephanie has learned that, given the choice, she would rather have tasty fresh berries.

```
1 — ②
1 — ③      ② — 3
① — 4      ② — 4      ③ — 4
1 — ⑤      2 — ⑤      3 — ⑤      4 — ⑤
1 — ⑥      ② — 6      3 — ⑥      ④ — 6      ⑤ — 6
```

FIGURE 4-C

Previously she put berries in the good-food category and ice cream and fudge on her bad-food list. Eating berries never seemed like having a choice because she felt no powerful intensity when she ate them. But when she ate chocolate fudge, because she had labeled it bad, her emotional reaction was rebellious pleasure and a lot of guilt.

When you do this grid, think of a time when you did something you felt was wrong, even if it was simple disobedience in childhood. Relax, perhaps close your eyes, and stay with the memory until you recapture that emotion.

Now transfer that same emotion to eating foods that you put on your bad list. If, for example, chocolate is a bad food and you eat it, you will likely *feel* you have done something bad.

When you ate a food you considered forbidden, did you feel guilty? Did you feel that you would have to punish yourself by denying yourself something or that you had already punished yourself by ruining your diet? Think about it for a few minutes and see if you can connect negative feelings with your eating. They are tied together more than most of us realize.

Now that you have done that, you can move beyond that emotional reaction to "hear" how your body is reacting to the food. Can you tell if you even like the taste?

When she ate chocolate fudge, because she had labeled it bad, her emotional reaction was rebellious pleasure and a lot of guilt.

See if you can connect negative feelings with your eating.

You build strength by unmasking your fear of food.

When you do this exercise, you build strength by unmasking your fear of food. As a result, you learn to think of food without self-recrimination.

For Stephanie, the berries were special, a pleasure to eat, but she didn't own that sense of specialness until she saw the choices in front of her.

Please remember, *Stephanie* made the choices, no one else. Because she was able to rely on what she wanted and move toward how her body reacted and the taste, the attitude that chocolate was addictive was disarmed and finally disappeared.

If chocolate had been Stephanie's first choice (it is for many of my clients), I would go a step further, saying, "Stephanie, tell me six different kinds of chocolate you enjoy."

Stephanie lists the following:

1. Häagen-Dazs chocolate ice cream
2. fudge chocolate
3. chocolate pie (French silk)
4. chocolate M&M's candy
5. chocolate-covered cherries
6. chocolate milk shakes

Stephanie and I go through the grid process again. (See 4-D.) Now her circles add up as follows:

```
1 — ②
1 — ③      2 — ③
1 — ④      2 — ④      ③ — 4
①— 5      ②— 5      ③— 5      ④— 5
1 — ⑥      2 — ⑥      ③— 6      4 — ⑥      5 — ⑥
```

FIGURE 4-D

1—1. Häagen-Dazs chocolate ice cream
2—2. fudge chocolate
5—3. chocolate pie (French silk)
3—4. chocolate M&M's candy

0—5. chocolate-covered cherries
4—6. chocolate milk shakes

When Stephanie prioritizes, her list comes out like this:

1. chocolate pie (French silk)
2. chocolate milk shakes
3. M&M's candy
4. fudge
5. ice cream
6. chocolate-covered cherries

———————————— □ ————————————

This exercise would show Stephanie, as it has shown many others, that not all chocolate is a problem. No matter how addicted Stephanie may feel, she knows she could leave the chocolate-covered cherries alone.

She might still insist, "But I'm addicted to chocolate pie."

So I would ask her, "If I said you can eat only chocolate pie for the next two weeks and nothing else, how would you feel?"

Her probable answer would be, "I'd tire of the pie. After a day or so, I'd want something else."

"That means you *like* chocolate pie; it's at the top of your taste preference. If you were truly addicted, you wouldn't tire of it. In fact, you'd want even more, more often and in larger amounts, because that's how true addictions work."

After they complete the grid, their fear of addiction disappears. They're more relaxed and calm toward chocolate or any food. "I'm not addicted to chocolate," they usually say with a surprised smile. "I just like chocolate." There's a world of difference; "like" doesn't wear a fright mask.

"If you were truly addicted, you wouldn't tire of it."

"I'm not addicted to chocolate," they usually say with a surprised smile. "I just like chocolate."

———————————— □ ————————————

I work from inside, allowing Stephanie to make her own choices. When she made the choices, she established her boundaries. I didn't say,

■ "Don't eat pie! It's too high in fat." (The attraction for chocolate would still be there.)

- "You may have one piece of chocolate pie a month." (I would be the permission giver, an external control, and the conviction of being addicted to chocolate would still be there.)
- "If you eat a lot of chocolate pie, you'll upset your nutrition and not be eating a healthful diet." (Aside from making her feel guilty, I wouldn't do anything toward alleviating her fear of addiction to chocolate.)

With the appropriate information and a few tools you can make choices and decide exactly where you want to set your boundaries.

I hope you understand the basics of the Inner Eating process. You learn to develop your internal boundaries. With the appropriate information and a few tools you can make choices and decide exactly where you want to set your boundaries. Inner Eating takes a little effort on your part, a little getting used to, but in the end it's worth it because *you* are worth it. You learn to be responsible for your decisions to take care of your body, like yourself more, and enjoy life more.

CHAPTER SUMMARY

You need a limited amount of nutritional information to make informed choices. The four food groups are meat, milk, bread and cereal, fruit and vegetable. Food choices strengthen your boundaries while restrictions create fear and rebellion. You label foods good and bad, eliminate the bad ones, and then crave them.

Fat in food serves the function of taste and satiety. The litmus test of food choice is how your body feels after you eat. Using circles helps overcome labeling and restricting. You can limit and define indulgences before you begin by using the circle concept. A grid exercise will help you sort out the foods you enjoy and label good or bad.

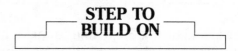

STEP TO BUILD ON

Make a grid for yourself. Select six foods you like, and go through each of the steps.

NOTES

1. Covert Bailey, *The Fit-Or-Fat Target Diet* (Boston: Houghton Mifflin, 1984), pp. 8, 14.

2. Paul Saltman, Joel Gurin, and Ira Mothner, *The California Nutrition Book* (Boston: Little, Brown and Company 1987), p. 109.

3. Henry Cloud, *When Your World Makes No Sense* (Nashville: Oliver-Nelson Books, 1990), p. 119.

4. Ellen Ruppel Shell, "Why You Always Have Room for Dessert," *American Health,* March 1986, p. 49.

5. Saltman, Gurin, and Mothner, *The California Nutrition Book,* pp. 37–38.

6. I'm indebted to James R. Sherman for the concept of the grids, which appears in his book *Rejection* (Golden Valley, Minn.: Pathway Books, 1982).

Rating Your Hunger

"I had the feeling that if I didn't hurry and grab a piece of pizza, I might not get another one."

Once a week Martha Wood and several other teachers went out for pizza. After one such outing, Martha said, "I had the feeling that if I didn't hurry and grab a piece of pizza, I might not get another one." She ate four pieces, far more than she really wanted to eat. "Why would I eat all those pieces of pizza?"

Because I wanted Martha to figure it out for herself, I asked, "What were you feeling while you were eating the first piece?"

"That I'd better hurry up and eat this one so I could get a second one."

"Okay," I said. "How did you feel when you were eating the second piece?"

"I was thinking I might like a third piece of pizza."

"What did you think during the third piece?" I asked.

"I know I'm going to eat a fourth piece of pizza so I might as well just do it."

As she started to reach for her fourth piece, she saw that only one slice remained on the platter. Martha turned to the teacher sitting next to her. "Would you like this last piece?"

"No, thanks," she answered, "I've had two, and that's really enough for me."

Martha ate her fourth piece, but she admitted, "I didn't enjoy it."

"When you finished that last slice of pizza," I said, "what did your stomach feel like?" That was the crucial question for Martha.

She thought for a moment before she said, "It felt stuffed."

You don't think about stopping; it doesn't occur to you that you can stop.

Although your experience may be somewhat different, you probably understand Martha. Like her, you don't plan to overeat, but you just keep on eating as long as food is available. You don't know how to stop yourself. Or you don't think about stopping; it doesn't occur to you that you can stop.

To help Martha understand her overeating, I showed her the Hunger Rating Scale. (See 5-A.) It will help you, too. As you can see, starving is 0, normal hunger is 2, and so it progresses through 10—which is being so full you may actually feel sick.

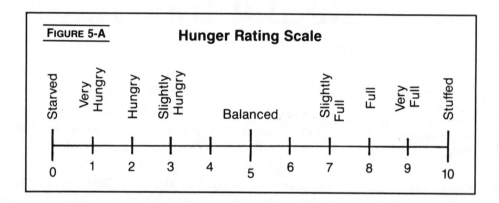

For example, let's say it's time to eat lunch, and you're down to a 4. This means you're not feeling particularly hungry when you and your friends go to lunch. What can you do?

The 5 is different for every person, so the scale doesn't impose a set rule.

You're aware that your slight feeling of hunger recommends that you order a light lunch to bring you up to a 5—and only you know when you reach 5. This scale shows the spectrum, but feelings are individual. The 5 is different for every person, so the scale doesn't impose a set rule.

I don't say, "Eat only when you're hungry." Such a rule just wouldn't work

- if your company had a prescribed lunch hour.
- if you had fifty minutes between appointments.
- if you're on a plane between Chicago and New York and you're served a meal.

You can't always wait until you're hungry to eat, although that's ideal. You may not have freedom with your schedule. If you're hungry at 10:45 A.M. but don't get a lunch break for another seventy-five minutes, you can't take time easily to eat. The time is already set for you; nevertheless, you can set the amount you eat.

I can already hear someone exclaim in disgust, "If I could control the amount of food I eat, I wouldn't need to read this book!" Don't get discouraged. Control isn't the issue; choice is. Right now I'm stressing that you can learn to choose the amount you eat.

Control isn't the issue; choice is.

On this 10-point scale, you've decided you're at 4, so you order a small lunch. If you were all the way down to a 1, you may want to eat a little more. Each time you eat, you decide where your body is on this scale.

NOTE TO MYSELF

I can stop eating when I choose.

When you reach the balance point, you stop eating. That's your goal. This balance point may be difficult for you to identify, especially in the beginning. It is for most of us because hunger is confused with so many other issues, and you're not used to making that kind of decision. On a diet you don't have to think about such issues. Maybe you eat half a grapefruit or three ounces of chicken and drink your flavored liquid. You're not encouraged to consider your individual need.

Hunger is confused with so many other issues.

The balance point is the neutral zone of eating. That's where you remind yourself to Stop! You're not on the starving to hungry side (0–3), and you're not on the full-to-stuffed side (7–10). You're absolutely balanced between the two extremes.

I can't describe how your balance point will feel to you; you will discover that for yourself. How do you determine the stopping point? Some of my clients speak about it this way:

- "It's where you feel satisfied."
- "When you're barely comfortable, but not too comfortable, you're there."

- "When I get the feeling that says I've had enough."
- "When my mind is at peace about what I've eaten."
- "When I feel energized from the food—not bogged down."
- "When my clothes don't feel tight when I have finished eating."
- "When my body feels so good about the amount of food I've eaten that I can enjoy the people I'm with—and not be obsessed with thinking that I ate too much food."

Once you experience the feeling and stop eating at the balance point, you'll be aware of the comfort.

To know this feeling for yourself, keep the Hunger Rating Scale in mind when you eat. Once you experience the feeling and stop eating at the balance point, you'll be aware of the comfort, and you'll build on the good feeling. Each time you have an eating occasion, you have an opportunity to practice eating to the balance point.

NOTE TO MYSELF

My balance point is where my meal gives me energy but doesn't make me sluggish.

Now I am going to give you another tool for applying the Inner Eating process: rating your circles of containment. To the left of the circle, place a number from the Hunger Rating Scale (p. 90) that rates how your stomach feels before you begin eating. To the right of the circle, put the number that rates your fullness when you stop eating. (See 5-B.)

Where do you usually find yourself when you close a circle of eating? Does the circle hold so much that you feel stuffed? Do you feel you are eating too much, but you keep on anyway? Do you say, "This food tastes too good to stop"?

The numbers on Martha's circle of eating indicate how her stomach felt before she started eating the pizza (left of circle) and when she ended (right of circle). (See 5-C.)

The time Martha Wood told me about eating four pieces of pizza, I asked, "Do you like pizza?"

"Oh, yes!"

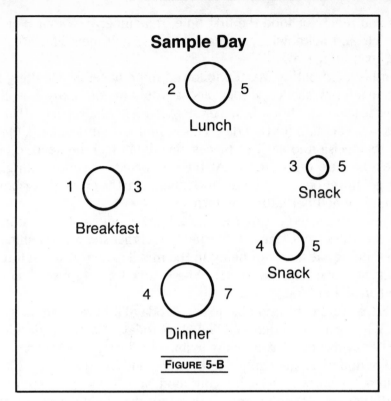

Sample Day

2 ◯ 5
Lunch

3 ◯ 5
Snack

1 ◯ 3
Breakfast

4 ◯ 5
Snack

4 ◯ 7
Dinner

FIGURE 5-B

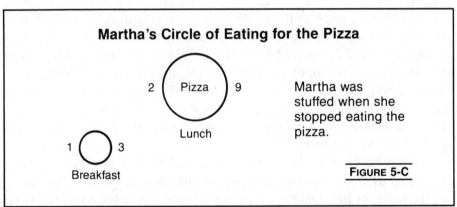

Martha's Circle of Eating for the Pizza

2 ◯ 9
Pizza
Lunch

Martha was stuffed when she stopped eating the pizza.

1 ◯ 3
Breakfast

FIGURE 5-C

"How many pieces would you have needed to eat to feel comfortably satisfied? To reach your balance point?"

"Probably two."

"Try this the next time you go out for pizza with the other teachers:

when you reach for food the first time, remember how four pieces of pizza felt and acknowledge what your stomach feels like after one piece, then after two."

On her next outing Martha followed my advice. By thinking how her stomach felt, she knew four pieces would be too many. She chose two pieces and identified how her stomach felt. She realized that two pieces were enough for that day. This is an important concept: Martha made the decision to eat two pieces. She didn't feel the need to hurry so she'd be sure to get more. At the end of her circle of eating, she didn't get upset because she ate too much. Martha created her boundaries and owned her eating pattern.

Martha made the decision to eat two pieces. She didn't feel the need to hurry so she'd be sure to get more.

When she started eating the pizza, Martha enjoyed the first piece. As she ate the second one, she started to feel that she was reaching the point of being satisfied—of being in the middle zone. After eating the second slice, she decided to stop. She enjoyed eating more than she had when she ate four pieces.

After eating the second slice, she decided to stop.

Martha has since been able to say, "Today I'll have salad instead of pizza." Or she'll say, "I think I'd like pizza today." Martha is learning to make her own choices. Not by my telling her, but by allowing herself to create boundaries, she can judge how her body feels.

Martha is learning to make her own choices.

Although you want to enjoy your food, you also want to enjoy your body. If the taste of food is more important than how your body feels, you may usually overeat to satisfy your taste. Learning to respect how your stomach feels is the best way to determine your balance point.

If the taste of food is more important than how your body feels, you may usually overeat to satisfy your taste.

Martha was influenced by the taste of the pizza, which caused her to overeat, but by understanding her balance point, she could have pizza without overeating. The issue of taste was combined with the issue of deprivation in a study to show why it's essential to make choices about taste rather than fear taste or punish yourself for wanting certain tastes and variety.

The study, done at Yale University,[1] worked with two groups. One group had an issue with weight—either overweight or underweight—but the other group did not. Those who had an issue with weight were more sensitive to the taste of food and could discern various tastes more readily than the other group.

Those who had an issue with weight were more sensitive to the taste of food and could discern various tastes more readily than the other group.

But the more interesting part of the study dealt with food deprivation. What happened when each group was deprived of tasty foods? The weight-issue group binged; the nonissue group did not. That demonstrated that the worst thing to do for persons who are sensitive to taste and have a weight problem is to deprive them of taste, as most restrictive diets do.

For those of us who love the taste of food, the study illustrates that if we deprive ourselves of tasty foods, we are in danger of bingeing. Thus, we may learn to fear tasty foods. We may never feel relaxed around food, always afraid that if we start to eat, we won't be able to stop. And if we don't stop and we really overeat, we may develop bulimia. On the other hand, if we keep eating everything that tastes good, which may have lots of fat in it, we may retain extra weight.

If we deprive ourselves of tasty foods, we are in danger of bingeing.

How can we live with such frustration? We don't have to. If we don't deprive ourselves of the food that tastes so good, and if we develop boundaries—Start! and Stop! limits—we can eliminate the problem.

That's easier said than done, I heard someone say. But instead of being afraid of it, take charge of it. Just knowing that you are more in tune to the taste of food, and that if you deprive yourself, you may binge, will help you understand how your body functions.

Instead of being afraid of it, take charge of it.

The more you learn about the natural harmony of your physical self and your mental self, the more you will diminish the behavior you don't understand or want. You will work as a harmonious whole being.

Deprivation comes in other forms, too, such as poverty. During the years of the Great Depression, Annie Laurie said that she and her parents went to bed many nights with empty, aching stomachs. "Even today when I sit down at a table, inside my head I have this feeling that I might not have another meal like this again. I'd better eat all I can get." And she does. Unfortunately, she taught this deprivation mentality to her children—quite unconsciously—and none of them would think of going to sleep at night on a scale of 2 or even 3. Annie Laurie overate at each meal because of the remembered fear of not having enough to eat. (See 5-D.)

"Even today when I sit down at a table, inside my head I have this feeling that I might not have another meal like this again. I'd better eat all I can get."

Deprivation can come from diets. If you're on a diet and stick to it, you may feel that you're starving, that you're never full, but you stay with the program. By staying slavishly with the diet plan, you ignore, or deny, the feelings of your stomach. If your stomach communicates, "I'm hungry," you fight the urge to eat because it's not time to eat. You're accepting the external boundaries of the diet—and fighting against your body.

Eventually you rebel and want variety and taste, and you break

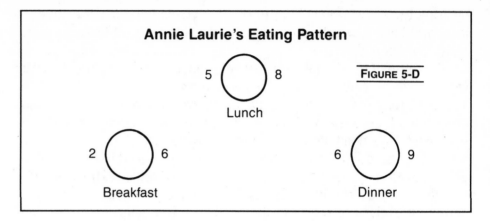

Annie Laurie's Eating Pattern

FIGURE 5-D

down the external boundaries. Because you haven't known how to listen to your internal signals, after days or weeks of deprivation, your body says, "No more!" You eat and overeat. (See 5-E.)

Meal skipping is another form of deprivation that can cause erratic meal patterns and distort your day's eating pattern to the point of severe discomfort and ultimate overeating.

Does the following situation fit you? You think, *I won't eat lunch today; I'll save the calories.* About two o'clock, the thought occurs, *I didn't have lunch, so I can have just a little bit.* That's when you begin nibbling.

Two important things happened.

1. You started out with the mind-set of not eating.
2. Because it wasn't a full meal, it didn't register as eating.

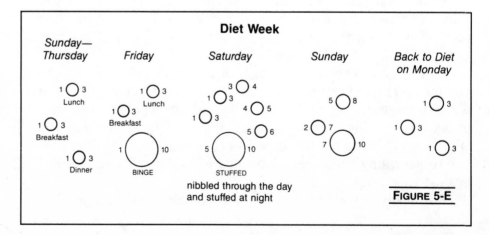

Diet Week

FIGURE 5-E

Unfortunately, snacking of small amounts usually continues, and you consume more than if you had stopped at noon for a regular meal. You also cheated yourself out of the real enjoyment of food. You never said to yourself, "I'm going to eat and enjoy my food." (See 5-F.)

Martha also told me of her problem with food in the teachers' lounge. Frequently people bring in food, and leave it out for the others to enjoy. "Anything left there is going to get eaten," she said, "just because of things like the stress of the day, the confinement of the buildings, knowing that you don't really go out. A trip to the lounge gives us a few minutes for relaxation."

One day somebody brought in muffins. "By the end of the afternoon," Martha said, "I had eaten four."

"How did you go about eating those four muffins?" I asked. "Just standing there, eating one after another?"

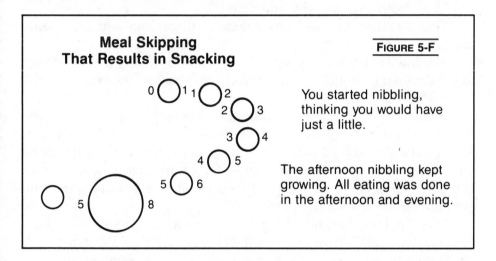

Meal Skipping That Results in Snacking

FIGURE 5-F

You started nibbling, thinking you would have just a little.

The afternoon nibbling kept growing. All eating was done in the afternoon and evening.

"Oh, no, of course not," she said.

"Tell me what happened."

Martha walked into the lounge, saw the muffins, and took one. She decided to eat half of it before returning to her classroom. Instead, she ate the whole muffin. Later she returned to the lounge and took a second one. Between classes, she went into the lounge again for "just one more." That time she ate two. After realizing she had eaten four muffins altogether, she was feeling ashamed and guilty.

"Could you have taken all four muffins, put them on a plate, and eaten them?"

After realizing she had eaten four muffins altogether, she was feeling ashamed and guilty.

"No, I wouldn't have wanted that many."

"If you had eaten them one after the other, how many muffins would have felt satisfying to you?"

"One. Maybe two." She admitted that she had started out thinking she was only going to eat "a couple of bites."

"Here's what I think happened," I said. "You never got into the act of eating. You didn't deal with eating the muffins as a circle. The eating didn't have a beginning and an ending. You never owned the circle of eating. You told yourself you were just going to munch at the circle. You never admitted to yourself, 'I'm going to eat.' So you kept nibbling until you ate four. By then you asked yourself how you could possibly have eaten so much."

The eating didn't have a beginning and an ending.

"That's right," she replied, "and you know, I didn't really enjoy eating them."

"Can you figure out why you didn't?"

"Now I realize it's that I never decided to eat four. I just kept eating."

"Putting it in my terminology," I said, "would you say that since you didn't consider the muffins a circle, you didn't contain the experience?"

Martha nodded.

I then suggested that if the situation occurred again, she could ask herself, How many muffins do I think would be satisfying? If two is her answer, she should take two. If she wants to munch on them throughout the day, that's a conscious choice. By eating that way, she could contain each circle of eating—that is, count it as a beginning and an ending. She could own it!

At any point in her munching, Martha could ask herself, How does my stomach feel? Where am I on the Hunger Rating Scale now?

Martha never thought she was going to nibble throughout the day. She kept thinking, *I'll have just a little.* But a little turned into a lot. (See 5-G.)

By drawing the circles and rating how your stomach feels at the beginning and ending of the eating occasion, you are making an effort to be honest with yourself about how often you eat for hunger.

———————————— □ ————————————

Do you eat the same way Martha did with the muffins? You nibble, but your actions simply don't register? When you start, you think, *I'm not going to eat anything much, just a bite or two.* And you actually overeat before you finish.

It comes down to a matter of saying, "I'm really not eating, I'm just nibbling" versus "I'm going to eat." When you stop trying not to eat and start owning your eating, your intentions are clear. That's why the circles and their ratings are important.

When you stop trying not to eat and start owning your eating, your intentions are clear.

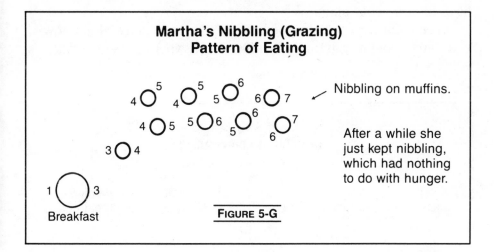

Martha's Nibbling (Grazing) Pattern of Eating

Nibbling on muffins.

After a while she just kept nibbling, which had nothing to do with hunger.

Breakfast

FIGURE 5-G

Skipping the meal isn't the issue. The important thing is the effect of meal skipping on your clear intentions to eat. I want to impress on you the significance of owning your decision to eat and assessing how your body reacts.

On the other hand, some people wait too long to eat. They won't eat breakfast because they have the idea that as soon as they start, they can't quit. They skip meals and later binge instead of nibbling. When you allow yourself to get really starved, you're most apt to feel out of control and overeat until you're stuffed.

When you allow yourself to get really starved, you're most apt to feel out of control.

If you're always battling hunger, you may consider hunger your enemy. Hunger isn't an enemy; hunger is a friend that informs you that your body requires fuel. If you deny the message, ignore the feeling, and fight hunger as your mortal enemy, you'll lose the battle or damage your body. Hunger, when denied and delayed long enough, will go on the attack.

Hunger is a friend.

Bear this in mind. When you feel the need to overeat, you may have waited too long to eat. You start at 0 on the scale, and you eat rapidly, without thinking about the feeling of your stomach. When you quit, you are at 9 or 10. (See 5-H.)

You may have been living this way a long time. You can't change your eating habits overnight. But you can do it.

Overeating can be induced by the Clean Plate Club ploy. If there's food in front of you, you have to finish it. You may recognize that you've reached a 5 on the scale, but you don't stop because you still have food on your plate.

When you were a child, you probably had no choice. Right now, if you think about it, you might be able to hear your mother's or father's voice saying,

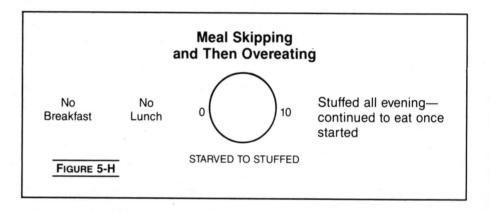

Meal Skipping and Then Overeating

No Breakfast   No Lunch   0   10   Stuffed all evening— continued to eat once started

STARVED TO STUFFED

FIGURE 5-H

- "Eat everything on your plate."
- "Don't waste food."
- "Somewhere in the world people are starving."
- "When you waste food, you waste money."
- "People in China (or South America or Asia) are going to bed hungry tonight." (One woman remembered saying to her father, "Then send the extra food to them!")

Put very small portions on your plate. You'll be surprised how little food you need to feel satisfied.

Teaching people that it's all right to leave food on their plate isn't easy because it's an emotional issue and hard for them to accept. One of those liberating facts for you may be the ability to say, "I can quit eating while I still have food left on my plate. It's not going to help or hurt anyone but me." And you can learn to do that! But if it's a seemingly impossible lesson to learn, put very small portions on your plate. You'll be surprised how little food you need to feel satisfied and how much money you can save on groceries in a year.

I believe there would be less waste of food if we got more in tune with our bodies. If we understand that we need only a certain amount to satisfy us, we would

- buy less at the grocery store.
- prepare less food at home.
- order less in a restaurant.

Rating each circle on the Hunger Rating Scale helps clients to assess the eating pattern relative to the degree of hunger. Placing the numbers to the left and right of the circle makes clear that they chose to eat right then and determined how their stomachs felt at that moment. By having their minds and stomachs working in concert, they are further encouraged to own their act of eating. (See 5-I.)

MEALTIME MESSAGES

These are messages that may be going through your head as you eat. Transfer the messages from your head to your stomach. Allow yourself to walk away from the food when you reach your balance zone. (See 5-J.)

"It tastes so good." (Counter with "My body feels good when I've eaten just to the balance zone.")

"I might not be able to get this food again." (Counter with "If I'm hungry, I can eat this again tomorrow.")

"I must clean my plate. I can't waste this food." (Counter with "Next time I need to be more aware of how much food my body needs when I'm this hungry. Then I won't order so much.")

┌─**NOTE TO MYSELF**─

How frequently I eat is my choice. I choose what works best for me.

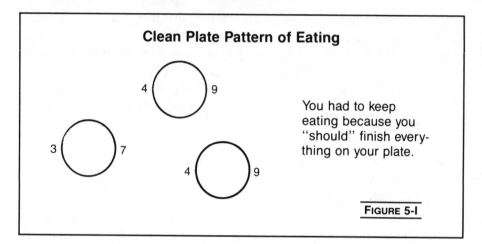

Clean Plate Pattern of Eating

4 9

3 7

4 9

You had to keep eating because you "should" finish everything on your plate.

FIGURE 5-I

Every time you have an eating occasion, stop eating when you're no longer hungry.

Every time you have an eating occasion, stop eating when you're no longer hungry. If you move beyond that, don't punish yourself. Be kind to yourself. Check the comfort level of your stomach. Don't listen to the familiar negative chatter in your head. Feel the discomfort if you're uncomfortable. Feel the fullness and know that you can choose not to feel that again.

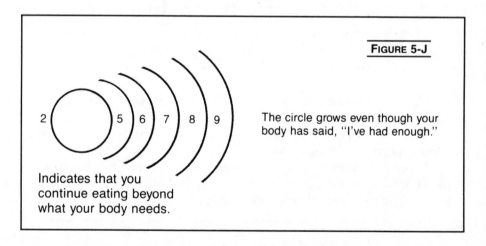

FIGURE 5-J

2 5 6 7 8 9

The circle grows even though your body has said, "I've had enough."

Indicates that you continue eating beyond what your body needs.

CHAPTER SUMMARY

Overeating can be a choice. The Hunger Rating Scale helps determine Start! and Stop! points to end overeating. A taste and deprivation study done at Yale University reveals that deprivation—such as a restrictive diet—is the worst way to deal with overweight persons. Creating internal boundaries is the solution to overeating. Meal skipping can lead to nibbling, snacking, and overeating because the act of eating isn't owned. Evaluating meals with the Hunger Rating Scale teaches sensitivity to hunger.

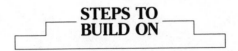

STEPS TO BUILD ON

1. Review the Hunger Rating Scale on page 90 to become comfortable with rating your own degree of hunger.

2. Familiarize yourself with the practice of placing numbers to the left and right of your eating circles to estimate where you began eating and where you stopped.

3. Consider the role that taste or food deprivation has played in your past eating pattern and determine the adjustments that are right for you.

4. If you're skipping meals, think about whether it's affecting your clear intention to eat.

NOTE

1. Richard E. Nisbett, "Taste, Deprivation and Weight Determinants of Eating Behavior," *Journal of Personality* 107–16.

Activity

6

Eating Becomes Something Else

I rushed home after a tennis game because I had to take care of an important business matter. Immediately upon entering the house, I walked directly to the cupboard. As I looked at the food on the shelves, it occurred to me, *I'm using food as a transition.*

Then came a second thought, *That's how I usually make the transition from recreation to business.* I also became aware that I wasn't the least bit hungry. I was using food to fill a need other than hunger.

I was using food to fill a need other than hunger.

That began my inquiry into unaware eating, the eating I was doing without thinking about it first. That led to my realization that sometimes eating serves a purpose other than providing the nutrition necessary to maintain a healthy body.

1. Eating as Transition

Even looking out the window would have worked, but for me, the habitual transition had become eating.

When we change activities, our bodies—heart rate, respiration, and even biorhythm—need time to catch up with our speedy brains, and food becomes an easy, convenient in-betweener. Until I thought through this matter of a transition period, I assumed that I moved from activity to activity to activity to activity to activity, with nothing else happening in between. Then I realized that I needed a break, perhaps only a short one, before I could refocus. Even looking out the window would have worked, but for me, the habitual transition had become eating—something, anything.

Using food as the intermediate activity made sense to me. (See 6-A.) Don't all people eat when they walk in the door? As far back as I could recall I had made my transitions that way. I might have let it go at that, except Jon came home while I was still pondering the idea. I decided to watch what he did between activities.

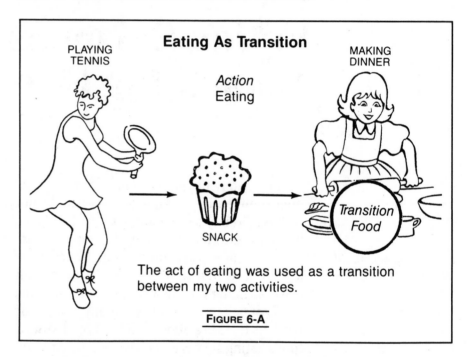

Eating As Transition

PLAYING TENNIS

Action
Eating

SNACK

MAKING DINNER

Transition Food

The act of eating was used as a transition between my two activities.

FIGURE 6-A

Jon kissed me, chatted a few minutes, and then went into the bedroom to change clothes so that he could work in the yard. As soon as he changed clothes, he went outside with no stopover in the kitchen. *Why doesn't he eat?* I wondered. The answer was obvious, but I didn't want to see it, so I continued to puzzle over the matter.

When Jon finished working outside, he came into the house, cleaned up, and sat down to read the newspaper. I couldn't believe it. My husband had been home for nearly two hours, and he still hadn't eaten anything.

"Jon," I asked, unable to stand it any longer, "why didn't you eat something when you came in from work? Or after you finished outside?"

Jon answered, "I didn't want to eat."

"But why?"

"Why should I?" he shrugged. "I wasn't hungry." He returned to his newspaper.

That afternoon's experience opened my eyes to how frequently some of us use eating as the break between activities.

Bill Thomas operated the way I did. As soon as he walked into the house after work, he headed for the kitchen and a cookie. From there he moved to the family room.

For me, for Bill, for thousands of others, this is a habit, an unconscious ritual of transition. Eating then becomes something else, something other than responding to hunger.

If you are currently using eating as a transition activity, as I did, you have a wide range of options to choose from. Even standing at a window and looking out for a couple of minutes is a possibility, and a healthy possibility, because it gives both mind and eyes a break without taxing the body.

When clients consider making the change, drinking water is often one of the first options that they think of, but then they ask if that isn't just continuing the oral habit of putting something in their mouths as transition. Well, yes and no, I tell them. Yes, it's oral, but on one hand, we are such an oral species that instinctively we want to put something in our mouths every ninety minutes. Drinking water is a pretty harmless way to satisfy that instinct and freshen the breath at the same time. On the other hand, all of the inhabitants on this water-based planet need a lot of water, and humans commonly don't drink enough water. Just plain water. Our bodies require it for optimum health. So, bottom line, I tell them to go ahead and drink water. It's a fine choice.

Drinking water is a pretty harmless way to satisfy that instinct and freshen the breath at the same time.

NOTE TO MYSELF

I will eat for hunger and enjoy it.

One client asked, "What else can you use for transition?"

Just let your body relax until you're ready to go again.

"Good question," I answered, because that had been the obvious question I'd asked myself. "The hardest and the easiest answer is also the simplest: just let your body relax until you're ready to go again."

"You mean just sit?"

"That's right."

"But what would I do with my hands?"

"Relax them," I said and chuckled because I had known only too well how difficult that simple answer was for her. "You're like so many of us. Our society teaches us to be busy every minute of the day. But who said we have to be doing something all the time?"

We emphasize doing, being productive, and getting results.

The German word *fleissig* means "industrious and hardworking." If you want to compliment someone, my German friends tell me, use *fleissig* in reference to her. In America, we're not much different because we emphasize doing, being productive, and getting results.

┌─**NOTE TO MYSELF**──────────────┐

It's okay for me to relax.

└────────────────────────────────────┘

2. Eating as Environmental Response

You eat by responding to the situation in which you find yourself at that moment.

Some individuals seem to

- have no issue with food.
- have no emotional bonds with food.
- feel good about themselves.

You may even visualize the meat sizzling on the charcoal. You're hooked.

But when they see or smell food, they're drawn irresistibly to it. If you're an environmental eater, these examples may describe your behavior.

- You aren't thinking about food, but you walk near a hotdog stand, *see* the glistening sausage, and have to eat one right now.
- You've just gotten out of your car and you're walking into the house. You *smell* the steak on your neighbor's outdoor grill.

You may even visualize the meat sizzling on the charcoal. You're hooked.

▪ You're cooking, and as you work, you *touch* the food, which you vowed not to eat. But touch leads to *taste,* and you nibble.

If these situations sound familiar, one expert would call you an environmental eater and would summarize you like this:

If you see food, smell it, hear it, think about it, or it's simply available, you eat it. You are particularly susceptible to pressure from other people, advertisements, social events. Weight problems usually begin with a moderate gain in the 30s, then slowly add up. You tend to be an impulse eater and consume larger than average portions.[1]

Insulin research done at Yale University by Judith Rodin and others confirms the fact that some people say they gain weight from just looking at food. Rodin says that thinking about food, whether triggered by the smell or a magazine ad, can actually change the body at that moment to make some people hungry. The change comes from insulin, the body's fuel regulator. This hormone guides sugar and fat from the bloodstream into the body's cells. Muscle cells then use the fuel for energy while the fat cells store it. Rodin writes,

Thinking about food can actually change the body to make some people hungry.

Insulin affects the brain as profoundly as the body. The same hormone that dispatches your food tells you to eat. High insulin levels make you hungry, make you eat more and make sweets taste better.

Insulin, in fact, appears to have much more to do with appetite than your level of blood sugar does.[2]

(This research confirms the importance of creating a beginning and an ending in your mind as well as in the actual eating.)

———————————— ☐ ————————————

Here are other examples of eating because of the environment or situation in which you find yourself.

Your young daughter is eating a candy bar.

As you watch, you suddenly want a taste. Many parents have done a great deal of persuading to get "just a bite" of what their child has. You want it because you see it now and you observe your daughter's

You want to eat because you see the food.

obvious enjoyment. Remind yourself that the yearning for her candy bar is environmentally induced. You want to eat because you see the food.

You're standing by the hors d'oeuvre table at a party.

Just being there where you see and smell the hors d'oeuvres may break down your resistance. If you decide you want to eat from the table, do so. It's still your decision. More important, recognize when you begin and when you end eating.

In your house you prominently display a candy-filled dish.

You seem unable to walk past the candy unless you pause long enough to put a piece or two into your mouth. If you're a nibbler, you're environmentally stimulated by this sight. Be kind to yourself and put the candy dish out of sight until you're able to disconnect food and environment.

You are grocery shopping.

This is an open invitation for environmentally stimulated people. Supermarkets have researched how to display the items to appeal to your various senses, including free taste samples of new products.

If you're hungry when you enter the grocery store (at level 1 or 2 on the Hunger Rating Scale [see page 90], and especially if you don't have a shopping list, your response to the environment may overcome your plan not to eat in the store. I'd suggest you get your eating level up to 3 or 4 before you go inside. In fact, budget advisers recommend never shopping when you're hungry.

You are going to have a buffet meal.

The variety of food can overwhelm you and bring out all your anxieties. Until you've developed internal limits, each item seems to cry out, "I taste rich and wonderful. Take me! Take me!"

So what can you do if you're an environmental eater? You have to decide that you can create boundaries to your eating. Remind yourself by saying,

- ▪ "I'm in charge of my eating."
- ▪ "I choose what, when, and how much to eat."
- ▪ "I eat only until I'm satisfied."

Once you learn to set your inner boundaries, your confidence grows, and you learn to trust your eating decisions. No matter how much food surrounds you, the choice still lies with you.

If you're an environmental eater, here is a self-affirmation for you.

Be kind to yourself and put the candy dish out of sight until you're able to disconnect food and environment.

Budget advisers recommend never shopping when you're hungry.

┌─NOTE TO MYSELF─────────────────┐

My surroundings don't dictate my eating.

└──────────────────────────────────┘

3. Eating as Activity

You are doing something else instead of concentrating on the actual eating. The eating just becomes a motion. Suppose you're settled in a comfortable chair to read a book. On the stand next to you is a glass of iced tea and a bag of popcorn. You snack as you read. You're barely conscious of the eating and drinking. When this happens, eating becomes just a motion rather than a conscious act.

Eating may be a passive activity, such as snacking when you're bored. (See 6-B.) Or you suddenly find yourself at the cupboard eating food you don't even like. Each time you eat needs to be a conscious decision that says, "I'm going to eat. I eat to take care of my body."

Eating can be an active, truly enjoyable experience—so enjoyable that you continue to eat more than your body needs. That's when eating becomes an activity done for the purpose of pleasure or enjoyment. Certain foods create an eater's high because they trigger the

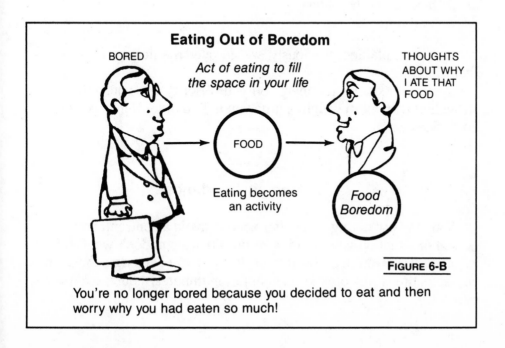

Eating Out of Boredom

BORED

*Act of eating to fill
the space in your life*

FOOD

Eating becomes
an activity

THOUGHTS
ABOUT WHY
I ATE THAT
FOOD

*Food
Boredom*

FIGURE 6-B

You're no longer bored because you decided to eat and then
worry why you had eaten so much!

production of endorphins—natural morphinelike painkillers in the brain.

Discover your favorite activity.

There's nothing wrong with seeking pleasure. You need it. Your body will seek it if you deny yourself endorphin-producing activities. Be responsible to yourself to find those pleasures. Endorphins are also released when you are in an activity you truly enjoy. Discover your favorite activity: dancing, reading, listening to music, walking, canoeing, gardening, skiing, playing tennis, going to the movies, taking nature hikes. Your personal endorphin-producing activity (or activities) will lead you away from eating-as-your-pleasurable-activity to much greater personal satisfaction.

When a client uses eating as an enjoyable activity, I usually work through the grid process with that person. (See chapter 4.)

"In addition to eating," I tell the person, "name five enjoyable activities."

The list might look like this:

1. eating
2. playing tennis
3. reading
4. gardening
5. talking on the phone
6. walking

As I've explained previously, we go over the items and prioritize them.

If eating becomes number 1 on your priority list, you'll always be struggling with extra weight. I urge you to find other things you love to do besides eat.

4. Eating as Avoidance

You may use eating as a buffer zone to avoid a confrontation with a person or situation you dread, a responsibility you don't want to face, an odious task you don't want to perform. If you eat long enough, you can sometimes put off the inevitable for minutes, hours, even days. (See 6-C.)

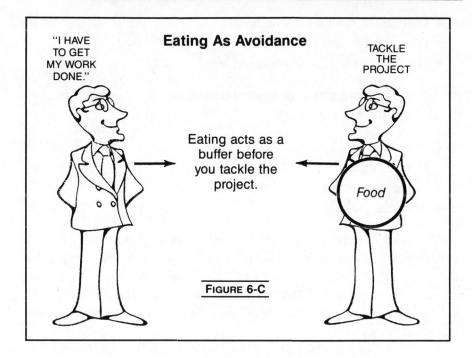

Eating As Avoidance

"I HAVE TO GET MY WORK DONE."

TACKLE THE PROJECT

Eating acts as a buffer before you tackle the project.

Food

FIGURE 6-C

5. Eating as Immediate Gratification

Immediate gratification was one of the toughest struggles for me because food reduced any strong emotions and satisfied my desire for results right now! It was if I said,

"I see it." - - - -> "I want it." - - - -> "I eat it."

No matter why we overeat, it always has the same result of unwanted pounds. We want those pounds off—and the faster, the better.

We live in an instant society, and we want everything fixed, healed, straightened, and arranged *now*. Diets remain popular because they offer immediate results. Think of the ads you've seen on TV about diet products; immediate success is a key marketing factor.

Diets remain popular because they offer immediate results.

Almost daily, TV commercials bombard us with a product that boasts, "Give us a week and we'll take off the weight." For years all kinds of magazines have proclaimed on their covers:

▪ Feel healthy without effort.
▪ Look ten years younger in ten days.

- Lose eight pounds in one week.
- Lose ten pounds before Christmas.
- Stop measuring, stop cooking; we'll do it for you.

All of these programs build on immediate appeasement. Immediate also means easy. It's easy

- to grab.
- to not prepare.
- to exert no effort.
- to avoid making decisions.

Those of us who work in the weight-loss field have become concerned about yo-yo dieters. Because so many live in the world of instant answers, they think if they can't lose twelve pounds in eight days, the diet isn't any good. Often they lose the weight and then go off the diet, only to have the weight sneak back on because they're not in tune with their bodies.

It takes time. You have to work at it.

I don't make promises about immediate results. The Inner Eating process offers no immediate gratification, but it does offer long-term help. I tell you how to help yourself. It takes time. You have to work at it.

I think of Linda who said, "I've got to lose some weight." No matter what I said, this idea remained uppermost in her mind. She was determined to lose weight now.

Linda has worked on a lot of issues in her life. Because she's bright, high-powered, and task-oriented, her single biggest problem concerned dealing with this matter of immediate results.

Through the exercise program, she lost inches, but the pounds came off gradually. Linda lost weight on almost every diet she tried—as long as she stayed on the diet. But a week off it and the pounds started to return.

Our society urges that luxury and success are signaled by abundance, but we must be thin—very thin.

In addition to immediate results, we live in a society of abundance where more is better and the more, the better. This concept transfers to food. Consider the variety of restaurants, from ethnic to fast-food. New kinds of food keep appearing in our grocery stores. Yet if we decide we must start eating smaller amounts, we think of deprivation. What a contradiction! Our society urges that luxury and success are signaled by abundance, but we must be thin—very thin.

You may be largely unconscious of the messages bombarding you every day. Yet you submit and subvert your personality to fit into the lifestyle around you. The act of eating, for instance, isn't done out of consideration for your body's needs. Instead, you eat to mold your body into the svelte look—or feel guilty because you can't.

Our media bombards us with thin models. We hear messages continuously about diet programs. One woman walked into my exercise class (a 7:00 A.M. class) and said, "Shirley, I have heard eight commercials on diets since I got up this morning at 5:00 A.M." Then the other commercials are about new and tasty food products! It's no wonder we have problems with eating issues in our country!

I'd like you to think of your eating as individual and separate from all of the promotions and advertisements and fads. Every year the rules change anyway, and if you learn to eat according to your body's needs, eating becomes personal, noncompetitive, and enjoyable.

If you learn to eat according to your body's needs, eating becomes personal.

As you work on clarifying the act of eating don't dig out and analyze all your peripheral problems first. However, if your issues block your ability to listen to your instincts, those issues need to be dealt with. If they aren't a block, don't magnify them. (See 6-D.)

EATING FOR AVOIDANCE

EATING FOR INSTANT GRATIFICATION

EATING AS A PLEASURABLE ACTIVITY BEYOND WHAT OUR BODY NEEDS

Healthy Act of Eating

EATING AS A TRANSITION

Eating for avoidance, instant gratification and transition were not big blocks for this person—and faded easily away when he concentrated on listening to and taking care of his body.

Eating as a pleasurable activity was a big issue for this person and needed to be dealt with. Finding other things to do that were more enjoyable than eating was the key to get rid of this block.

FIGURE 6-D

Let's see how this works by setting up a possible situation. For some time you've been listening to your body when you eat. You walk past a food stand and smell the caramel corn. Because your body is strong, the inner dialogue might sound something like this: *That sure smells good, but I'm just not hungry.*

He hit a roadblock, and the weight started to come back on. He couldn't figure out why.

Presently I'm working with a man I'll call Sam. He heard me speak at a meeting and the only thing he carried away was, "Eat only when you're hungry." Sam had tried several diets, but none of them worked. Just learning to eat only when he was hungry was enough so that, for the first time, he started to lose weight. Then he hit a roadblock, and the weight started to come back on. He couldn't figure out why.

He realized that he overate only at home.

After we talked at length, Sam began to isolate his eating pattern. He realized that he overate only at home. At work he was an efficient man who handled situations well. However, his wife has a strong, domineering personality. Rather than confront her on issues he didn't agree with, Sam started eating, avoiding the problem: eating as avoidance.

Once Sam became aware of this roadblock, he separated his eating from his situation. When he felt attacked at home, instead of reaching for food to avoid his feelings, he decided to find other ways to cope with the situation. (See 6-E.)

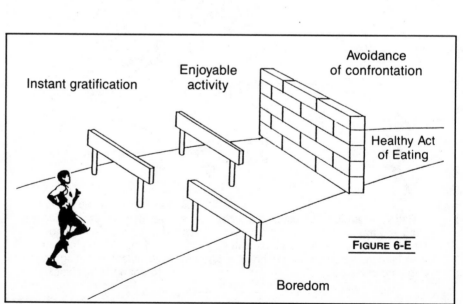

FIGURE 6-E

"Sam," I said, "see if it helps to think of it this way. You're walking calmly down a road. This is your eating awareness road. Everything is going fine until you see a roadblock ahead. What are you going to do? What are your options?"

"I could turn around and go back the way I came," he said, "but I wouldn't get anywhere." He suggested a few other possibilities before he decided he could simply remove the roadblock.

In practical terms, Sam chose not to eat because of the situation at home. He also decided he was going to learn to express his feelings instead of remaining silent. All he needed was to become aware that he had options.

All he needed was to become aware that he had options.

One solution Sam could have chosen was to think of every possible roadblock, get rid of them, and then start the trip. Then he realized, "This could take forever." If he concentrated on his journey, he would encounter blocks, but he could deal with them as he got to them.

If you choose this option, you allow your body to steer the course around the obstacles on the eating road. By your concentrated focus on the positive aspects of your journey, you find it's a pleasant and faster learning experience.

Ted Warner, a tennis pro, taught tennis in much the same way. His focus was to create the correct form through a positive statement rather than telling the student what he is doing wrong and trying to correct every error. He's careful not to say, "Don't swing your racket on the volley." He expresses the positive: "Nose, toes, and racket move together." There is a parallel in Inner Eating. Don't say, "Don't eat so much." Do say, "Eat to your balance point." Also, the eating for reasons other than listening to your body may gradually fade away if your focus is on the positive, respecting your body. You don't need to conquer every issue to stay on your path.

Don't say, "Don't eat so much." Do say, "Eat to your balance point."

CHAPTER SUMMARY

We use eating as a transition activity, as a response to our environment, as something to do—either as a passive endeavor or as an active search for pleasure—as a means of avoiding something, and as immediate gratification. Usually, focusing on the act of eating encourages other reasons for eating to resolve themselves. If it doesn't, the blocking issue needs to be confronted.

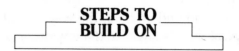

STEPS TO BUILD ON

1. Identify your eating-for-something-else occasions by seeing where you are on the Hunger Rating Scale when you begin or want to eat relative to your balance point. If you are a 5 or over, you are definitely eating for other reasons. Identify those reasons. (See 6-F.)

2. Determine why you began or continued to eat by answering the following questions:

Where was I when the trouble eating began?

How did I feel? Stressed, bored, tired?

How hungry did I feel?

When did I stop listening to my body?

3. List six other options to eating and make a grid.

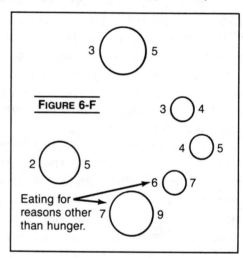

FIGURE 6-F

Eating for reasons other than hunger.

NOTES

1. Maria Simonson and Joan Heilman, "Johns Hopkins University Weight-Loss Plan," *Family Circle*, May 3, 1983, p. 55.

2. Judith Rodin, "Taming the Hunger Hormone," *American Health*, January/February 1984, pp. 43–44.

Achievement/
Perfectionism

7

Eating as Achievement

"Oh, you're s-o-o-o thin!"

"Jennifer, you did such a good job with your diet."

"How did you manage to lose all that weight and still look so good?"

Those are the kinds of comments Jennifer heard. And like anyone else in a similar situation, she enjoyed the attention and admiration. For her, the primary reason for losing weight became achieving a goal; achievement meant success.

She enjoyed the attention and admiration.

Losing weight became Jennifer's primary way of excelling and of being noticed. Unfortunately, when she got down to a weight that was good for her body, she had no signals to tell her to stop. She still wanted to achieve, so how could she stop the one thing that made her special?

Unaware of what she was doing to herself, Jennifer had linked weight loss to her sense of self-esteem. If she stopped shedding pounds, she stopped achieving, and that meant her self-esteem plunged. She kept getting thinner, and eventually she became anorexic. (Clinically, an anorexic is at least 15 percent below normal weight.)

Jennifer had linked weight loss to her sense of self-esteem.

Even though her doctor hospitalized her for anorexia, Jennifer didn't realize until much later that she "still felt that eating and achievement were linked because they kept telling me I had to eat. They kept setting goals for my weight."

Her achievement mentality hadn't changed; only now she was achieving weight gain instead of loss. Daily, people asked Jennifer the

People asked Jennifer the achievement question, which began, How much . . . ? or How many . . . ?

achievement question, which began, How much . . . ? or How many . . . ?

- How much have you eaten?
- How many times have you eaten?
- How much weight have you put on this week?
- How many total pounds have you gained?

At the hospital, everything seemed to center on achievement.

- The nutritionist laid out an eating plan for her—following it was the achievement.
- When she reached a certain weight, the doctor would release her—another achievement.
- The scales constantly measured accomplishments of the way her body looked, the success of her nutrition plan, and the number of pounds she should weigh.

The doctor's plan didn't change her achievement orientation.

Consequently, other than getting her to gain weight, the doctor's plan didn't change her achievement orientation. I started working with Jennifer after her release from the hospital. Her mother could see that although she was out of immediate physical danger, Jennifer remained obsessed with weight and food.

"Do you enjoy eating?" That's the first question I asked Jennifer. She stared back at me, silently, stunned by the question.

"What's wrong?" I finally asked.

"No one ever asked me that before," she said. "I never thought about whether I liked to eat. At least, I haven't for a long time."

As we talked, I realized that Jennifer was afraid to think of enjoyment because she linked food with pain, anger, and frustration. She feared that if she learned to like food, she would eat more, and that would make her fat.

"When you do something as intimate for yourself as eating," I said, "let it be your choice. As you continue to make these choices, you gain inner strength."

First, Jennifer had to disengage eating from achievement. Instead of emphasizing goals, I stressed the importance of making her own choices and gaining the inner strength that follows. Jennifer and I worked slowly at giving her back the right to make her own selections.

┌─ **NOTE TO MYSELF** ────────────────────┐

"The strongest principle of growth lies in human choice." —George Eliot

└──┘

Whenever Jennifer slipped back into the achieving cycle, I'd ask, "What would *you* like?" In the Inner Eating process, Jennifer began to listen to herself and to reclaim who she is.

Jennifer began to listen to herself.

Although it came about gradually, Jennifer chose to take care of her physical health. (See 7-A.) She didn't have an easy task because she had to learn to trust her body signals. Once she did, however, Jennifer started to discover things about herself. She could

- concentrate on the moment of eating.
- make her own choices.
- enjoy her body.
- relax when eating.

┌──┐

Path from Anorexia to Health

GOAL: *Thin Body*
1. Fear of Food/Fear of Eating
2. Mind/Body Unity Separated
3. Body As Achievement Tool

GOAL: *Physical Health*
1. Understanding Body's Use of Food
2. Awareness of Hunger Instinct
3. Physical Fitness

FIGURE 7-A

└──┘

Jennifer began to make progress, and she could see that her primary achievement had been a thin body. That was her comfortable and known achievement world, and she was the center of it. When she thought of eating for physical health instead of for a thin body, she recognized that she faced finding a new goal for herself. That realization frightened her. The risk of attempting something new and the fear that followed would sometimes throw her back to focusing on some part of her body that she could perfect, such as her derriere. She knew

She faced finding a goal for herself other than her thin body.

how to accomplish a thinner body. Jennifer worked hard at not falling back into the pattern of anorexia.

Jennifer knew she had to get out of her self-destructive pattern. To get unstuck, she needs tools to help her make choices today. The Inner Eating process, as discussed in previous chapters, offers tools for making choices about eating for physical health, such as learning to recognize hunger and fullness as well as the body's need for nutrition. Once Jennifer learns to make choices about eating and food and is comfortable doing so, she is equipped to transfer those skills to the larger arena of choices about her life goals, immediate and long-term. If she finds herself blocked at some point, needing assistance to develop career tools, for example, she can seek advice from another appropriate person.

Two dynamics that affected Jennifer's life—achievement and competition—were tied to the act of eating. All that together triggered anorexia. In addition, her sister was dieting successfully. Like many sisters, the two had competed all their lives, but Jennifer had been thinner. Only later was Jennifer able to figure out that she thought her sister was taking away her one area of accomplishment. She couldn't diet anymore; she was already too thin. Since the situation angered and frustrated her, falling back into competition could easily have destroyed Jennifer. Had she gone back to her old pattern of trying to outdo her sister, she might have killed herself.

"Jennifer," I said, "you need to see yourself as being separate from your sister." Because she didn't grasp immediately what I was driving at, I drew two stick-figure people with a circle around each. (See 7-B.)

Once Jennifer learns to make choices about eating and food and is comfortable doing so, she is equipped to transfer those skills to the larger arena of choices about her life goals, immediate and long-term.

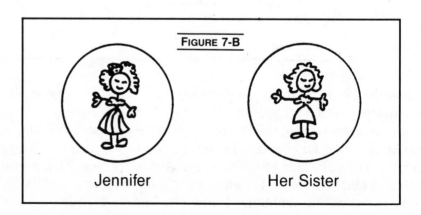

FIGURE 7-B

Jennifer   Her Sister

The circles enabled Jennifer to create her own boundaries because she could see her sister and herself as two separate people. She had been trying to out-thin her sister. Jennifer had to perceive herself as an individual and allow her sister to be whoever she wanted to be.

"You don't have to be thinner than she is to be acceptable," I said. "Just be you. You're acceptable as you are."

The two circles also helped Jennifer in her relationship with others because she frequently felt diminished around other people. She felt as if she lost a part of herself whenever she was with some individuals. Through extreme self-control, she was trying to reclaim possession of herself.

People who are empathetic, sensitive to others' needs and feelings, especially need healthy boundaries to avoid being pulled off center—to lose their focus—or to avoid being sucked dry—emptied of their emotional vitality. There are two common reactions to having one's boundaries overwhelmed: to starve to regain control of one's feelings of integrity, or to overeat to refill the resulting sense of emptiness. (See 7-C.) Inner Eating helps these people build healthy relationships by learning to make choices.

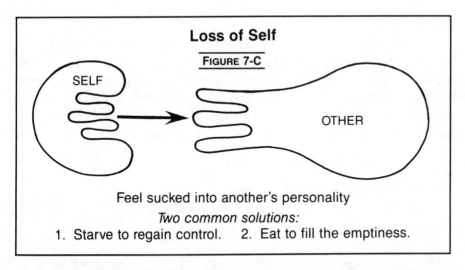

Loss of Self

FIGURE 7-C

SELF

OTHER

Feel sucked into another's personality

Two common solutions:
1. Starve to regain control.   2. Eat to fill the emptiness.

Jennifer would get this off-center feeling especially around her sister but with others, too. When she got away from them, she used starving as her way to regain control. In her early years, Jennifer ate when she felt invaded; the focus on food protected her core self. Later, concentrating on getting thinner, she didn't have to cope with those feelings. In either case, fat or thin, her focus on food became her way of coping with feelings of invasion.

Once Jennifer felt that her core self was safe, she could work on her misplaced focus on food and concentrate on being a whole person. Jennifer learned to eat. Yet for a long time, eating still translated into fear of getting fat, so she threw herself into frenzied exercise. "I felt that if I didn't exercise, the food was going to turn my body into something ugly and fat." Gradually she learned to connect the act of eating food with caring for her body.

Eating and achievement can get all mixed up in the mind, and a person may believe,

"I felt that if I didn't exercise, the food was going to turn my body into something ugly and fat."

- If I am fat, I am a failure.
- If I am thin, I am successful.
- If I am successful, I can be happy.
- To be successful and happy, I must lose weight. The more weight I lose, the more successful and happy I'll become.

———————————— □ ————————————

I recall reading an article with the title "A+ Achiever Gets F− in Weight Loss." The writer told my story without knowing it. The article bemoaned the fact that organized, high-achieving women who meet virtually every goal they set for themselves fail when it comes to losing weight. A research project conducted in Rochester, New York, involving 450 women was cited. They were women who

High-achieving women who meet virtually every goal they set for themselves fail when it comes to losing weight.

- hated wasting time.
- tended to rush through their tasks.
- thought about work during their off-hours.
- felt strongly competitive.

Yet those very women were frustrated with their diets because they expected too much, too fast. Dieting didn't yield to greater effort, like other tasks.

———————————— □ ————————————

Linda Kemp is a high-achieving, goal oriented woman who felt that she could set a goal of eating right to achieve the body she wanted. She says,

"In the past I dieted the way I did everything else, systematically, with my eyes on my goal, and doing everything correctly to solve the problem. I'd choose a diet and follow it perfectly. If it called for half a grapefruit, a bowl of cereal, and a cup of skim milk, that's what I'd eat.

"I'd choose a diet and follow it perfectly."

"Each diet was successful. I'm an authority on diets—I've been on more than twenty in my lifetime. I followed the diets faithfully and would lose between twenty and forty pounds, and then it would all come back on. After being on so many diets, my metabolism had adjusted, slowed down, so that I could go on a 500-calorie diet and still not lose weight. I was working against my body. What I needed to do was learn how to eat and exercise to get my metabolism up again.

"After being on so many diets, my metabolism had adjusted, slowed down, so that I could go on a 500-calorie diet and still not lose weight."

"Also, I realize that although I ate the foods and smaller amounts, I just followed the rules as a means of losing weight.

"When I first started working with Shirley, she talked about enjoying food. That was a fresh concept for me, and once I began, I found myself enjoying new sensations.

"Before that, I'd tell people I liked to eat, and that's why I ate a lot. Now I realize that I hadn't given food much thought, much less enjoyed it. I don't like to cook, and food wasn't a particularly important part of my life. But that doesn't mean that I didn't eat. I ate compulsively. If there was a box of cookies in the house, I didn't quit until it was gone.

"I ate compulsively. If there was a box of cookies in the house, I didn't quit until it was gone."

"I ate fast and thought about other things. One of the things I liked about being on a diet was that I didn't have to select my menu. I just followed someone's plan. I didn't have to waste my time thinking about what, when, or how to eat.

"In contrast, my husband truly enjoys eating good food, and he has no weight problem. When he sits down to eat a meal, he wants to eat it slowly and enjoy it. He savors the flavors. I, on the other hand, ate so fast that I didn't know what the food tasted like. He teased me by saying, 'You don't have to hurry. I'm not going to take your food away from you.'"

"I ate so fast that I didn't know what the food tasted like."

Linda laughs as she tells a story that illustrates how achievers will use their ingenuity to accomplish a diet's dictates.

"I'm not a hot dog eater. I've never, in fifteen years of marriage, fixed a hot dog for my husband. But once I was on a diet that called for hot dogs on the second night. I was on a business trip with another person at the time, and she decided to join me on the diet.

"When we reached our destination, we stopped at a market and bought our all-beef hot dogs, green beans, and beets. In our hotel room, we opened our canned vegetables with a can opener I carried and then looked around for a solution for a cold, unappetizing meal.

"I love a challenge. I called housekeeping and had them send up an iron, took the iron into the bathroom, and grilled our hot dogs on the bathroom countertop."

Linda has come a long way since then. She had to get beyond making weight loss her goal, her achievement, and to put it aside until she worked through other issues.

She had to get beyond making weight loss her goal.

Weight wasn't her primary problem—achievement focus was. Seeing that was hard, and dealing with it was even harder because the change needed to come from within. After six months of working through the Inner Eating process, she hadn't lost enough to suit herself, so she decided to take charge of the situation—she'd go on a diet.

But something happened that made her change her mind. As she was watching television with her husband, a diet plan commercial came on the screen. He looked over at her and said, "I'm so glad you don't do that dieting stuff anymore. You're much nicer and more fun to be around when you're not dieting. I think you must be getting to the core of Shirley's process now."

His comment helped her see that returning to diet thinking would only get her working against her body again. She decided to stick with the Inner Eating process, trust her body, and give it more time.

Working with the concepts of choice and enjoyment with eating has affected other areas of her life.

Linda has stayed with the Inner Eating process for almost two years now. She enjoys food more and eats less, and she doesn't eat compulsively. Her weight has maintained itself, and she is now starting slowly to lose weight. She still doesn't like to cook, she says with a laugh. Working with the concepts of choice and enjoyment with eating has affected other areas of her life, too. She has learned to identify other pleasurable activities, something she never thought of before.

Dieters, who are highly goal-oriented and like to be in control of their lives, tend to get frustrated when a weight-loss plan, even one that is healthy and realistic, doesn't produce results on their predetermined schedule. They can accept challenges in just about every other area of life but are unsuccessful in their own eyes in the area of weight control.

This is just as true for men who are taught to be goal oriented. Take away the achievement factor, and they find it difficult to cope. They ask,

- "If there's no goal, who am I?"
- "What's my purpose then?"
- "To lose weight, do I have to stop achieving?"

I'm not against goals and achievement. My concern is that you don't make it your goal to be thin at the expense of caring for your body. When you make thinness your goal, you can't hear your body signals because you're listening to another voice.

Like Jennifer, I had once considered eating to lose weight on the same level as any other achievement. I worked at it as a specific goal. As I've already pointed out, my husband, Jon, allowed me to observe eating as I'm convinced it was meant to be, to take care of the body, first, and to enjoy food, second. (See 7-D.)

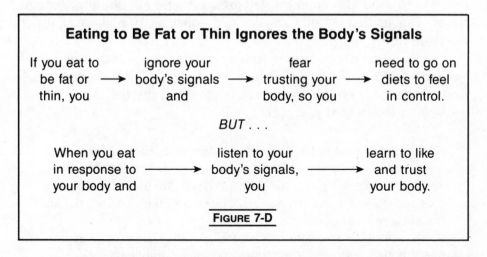

Eating to Be Fat or Thin Ignores the Body's Signals

If you eat to be fat or thin, you → ignore your body's signals and → fear trusting your body, so you → need to go on diets to feel in control.

BUT . . .

When you eat in response to your body and → listen to your body's signals, you → learn to like and trust your body.

FIGURE 7-D

The same year that Jon and I married, my teaching position was cut. Then I became pregnant. Things changed quickly from being a single, career person to an at-home wife and expectant mother.

Still caught up in the achievement cycle after Katie was born, I thought, *I'll work on my Ph.D. now.* However, one day while I was in class, my body demonstrated that it was time to feed Katie. I was a nursing mother, but she was at home and I was at the university.

I had to start making choices.

That's the day I realized I had to start making choices and setting priorities. After I had thought through all my options, I asked myself a few simple questions, such as,

- What's right for me?
- What are my short- and long-term goals?
- What do I want right now?

I chose to pull back from outside achievements. I would stay at home to give my time and energies to my daughter and my husband. But it wasn't as easy as I expected, and my new mother-wife choice didn't seem very exciting.

I was able to discover who I was without the external pressures.

Although I had to do some adjusting, I realize now that the time I stayed home with Katie, followed two years later by Steven's birth, was a wonderful experience for me. I was able to discover who I was without the external pressures of how well I was doing outside the home.

Besides that, I had the opportunity to observe more carefully Jon's reaction to food and eating. I gathered information on nutrition and fitness. During that period I also decided—once and for all—to conquer the issue of my weight.

I didn't want my body size to be an issue for the rest of my life. I wanted to like my body and to enjoy living in it. That's when I confronted the focus on the role of achievement in my life.

Colette Dowling says it well:

Good feelings tend to be attached to achievement and achievement only. Many of us have no idea what it's like to feel consistently good about ourselves. We go up and we come down. We use externals—our own accomplishments, the accomplishments of our children, the accomplishments of husband and friends—to try to boost ourselves. Rewards, approval, and admiration have become the ingredients of a magic potion with which we try to cure inner emptiness.[1]

The fortunes of body image have varied for women and men over the centuries. The male body image for the early Greeks was a significant cultural symbol. Corpulent meant rich, muscular equaled beauty, and thin revealed poverty. Thinness for women didn't become a rebellious ideal until the flappers kicked up their heels during the Roaring

Twenties. Now men have been snagged again by body image. They want to be thin but muscular, demonstrating their dual achievement of money enough to be healthy and leisure enough to be tanned and toned.

If you struggle with this image-achievement complex, you know how it works. When you feel the inner emptiness Ms. Dowling refers to, you eat when you are between achievement goals.

I had the chance to sit with my emptiness while I was off the external achievement track. Then one day I had a startling revelation: I felt my emptiness in the same place I felt hunger.

I had a startling revelation: I felt my emptiness in the same place I felt hunger.

"That's it! That's it!" I said. When I asked who I was, I felt an inner emptiness. I had learned early in life to fill that empty space with food. After I filled it, I had to worry only about the extra weight, not who I was, so I could avoid answering my question.

———————————— □ ————————————

The issue of achievement and eating and how it gets mixed up with image and self-esteem is vital for you to understand. I'll use my own story again as an example. As a young person, you'll remember, I had a history of steady achievement in many areas at one time. It wasn't something negative or destructive in my life or in my family's life; accomplishment was a joy to us all, individually and collectively.

However, when I became a wife and mother and discovered that the logistics of time and human energy meant I had to get off the achievement track and concentrate on my family, the only thing I had left to do was achieve through my children and my eating. Neither option was acceptable.

I was I, valid and whole and disinclined to be a Svengali to others I honored as valid, whole people, who didn't need me controlling them. Achieving through eating didn't work, either, because it created only frustration, which was so unlike any other achievement focus I'd ever known. I was stuck!

What I went through as a result of that impasse took several years and produced many revelations. At the core was the realization that working to achieve a thin body went against my instincts. I was at war with myself, and human instinct is to be in harmony with oneself.

Working to achieve a thin body went against my instincts.

I planned to return to my achievement track when I could, little knowing that even then I was achieving on an entirely new level. This one was internal—that's why I call it Inner Eating because the purpose is to separate eating for physical health from *all other issues*.

When you eat to control body image, health and vitality can get lost to the control issue. Achievement is a form of control, and eating and achievement get so tangled together that you lose the ability to hear or understand your body signals or instincts. And those signals and instincts keep you physically and mentally healthy.

Eating and achievement get so tangled together that you lose the ability to hear or understand your body signals.

Consequently, I learned and practiced with my clients that, first, whether you are overweight, anorexic, or bulimic, your primary mental aim is to separate eating from all other issues, such as body image and weight.

Extra eating has nothing to do with your body's needs.

Second, your body isn't responsible for your achievement or for defining who you are; your brain is your action center. Your extra eating has nothing to do with your body's needs. You can't eat to compensate for inaction or indecision. If you try to compensate in that way, your body gets padded and you're still stuck with inaction and indecision.

———————————— □ ————————————

When I saw that I could separate my physical hunger from my psychological hunger, eat in response to my physical hunger, and find other ways to take care of my emotional needs, something else became blazingly clear. I could accept myself for who I was and for where I was at that time. And I didn't need to achieve anything to do so. I was free to eat in response to how my body felt *at the moment*.

Previously I had been trying *not* to eat.
I ate to become thin.
I ate because the diet said to.
I didn't know any longer what hunger felt like.
I ignored my body's signals.

I became an artichoke, something I could peel to the heart.

My interior journey scared me. I felt that I was peeling myself like an onion, and one day I would get down to where there was nothing left. I would be gone. But then I saw that I was scaring myself with images. So I became an artichoke, something I could peel to the heart. There! That felt good. My heart, my core self, the essential me. I looked forward to finding my essence.

CHAPTER SUMMARY

Eating for weight loss, or thinness, links weight, self-esteem, and achievement. Anorexics are often high achievers whose thinness is an achievement orientation. Anorexics lose ability to read their body signals. Placing blame for anorexia is counterproductive. Help comes from gaining a renewed capacity to make choices and building healthy boundaries. Empathetic people can be drained by others' neediness, and they overeat or starve to regain their feelings of integrity. They need to reconnect the act of eating with hunger. High achievers have a hard time losing weight because they ignore their body signals. Emotions are often felt as hungerlike emptiness. The Inner Eating process separates eating from all other issues. The body isn't responsible for achievement or self-definition; the brain is. Feeding physical hunger and accepting yourself right now free you to respond appropriately to emotional needs.

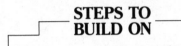

STEPS TO BUILD ON

1. I will listen to my body signals and try to separate my physical hunger from emotional hunger (emptiness). If I'm hungry, I'll eat.

2. I will be aware when other people's behavior invades my boundaries, and I will work to build healthy boundaries.

3. I will respect my physical health rather than use my body or my physical image as achievement.

NOTE

1. Colette Dowling, *Perfect Women* (New York: Pocket Books, 1988), pp. 30–31.

8

The Barrier of Perfectionism

"When I get thin, everything will finally be perfect."
"Why shouldn't I be the best at everything I do?"
"Why shouldn't I be perfect?"
"I'll work at a job until I can't do it any better."
"I look forward to a challenge so I can improve."
"If something is worth doing, it's worth doing perfectly."
Those are my words! I said them. I believed them. I had become a perfectionist.

My focus had been achievement, and I felt that I could accomplish anything I chose to do. No one had ever told me that I couldn't achieve, or that I didn't have the right, or that what I did wasn't good enough.

When I married a man who had definite, productive ways of doing things, he tried to help me learn to do them his way. I tried, because I liked how he did things. However, I gradually felt that I couldn't do things right on my own. My self-confidence was weakened. When I realized what was happening, I told Jon that we had to talk.

I told him that in my efforts to do things his way, I had become perfectionistic, and it was immobilizing me. I felt trapped because I feared failure, and I doubted myself. I wasn't sure I could achieve my chosen goals.

I had become perfectionistic, and it was immobilizing me.

Jon listened and understood. He hadn't meant to degrade me in any way. Then I realized I had made his suggestions into absolutes. Just as I knew choices in eating created strength, I needed to get back to making my own choices in life, although I could learn from others.

I didn't want to get stuck in an all-or-nothing bind.

Meanwhile, I had to work myself out of my perfectionism. I knew I wanted quality, but I could settle for something less than perfect. I didn't want to get stuck in an all-or-nothing bind. I had to think this through.

The creative part of me had frozen while I pushed to be perfect because creating is an imperfect process—at least for humans. I grew up in a home where I rarely heard "you can't" and "you shouldn't," so I had felt free to be creative in my approach to achievement. But then, when I worked to fit Jon's mold, I went from high expectations to high, perfect expectations, which created fear of failure.

I would trust myself to know my instincts best and not rely on others to set my goals for me.

However, I saw that I could choose quality and enjoy the process, the task, the journey. It was an internal shift, an attitude change that probably didn't show on the outside. It was a decision to do my best and be happy with it. I would trust myself to know my instincts best and not rely on others to set my goals for me.

"Okay, Shirley," I told myself, "apply that to your struggle with weight."

After some thought I recognized that our culture's image of how we should look was still causing me perfectionistic problems. I was amazed to see how I, a generally self-motivated person, got hooked by society's thin-body values. I had internalized that value at the expense of trusting my instincts.

THIN is in!
Only THIN is beautiful!
Only THIN is happy!
Only THIN is fun!
Only THIN is popular!
THIN is athletic!

We have sabotaged ourselves by believing that we have to be thin and we have to be perfect.

We're victims of media hype, a constant barrage of pictures that encourages us to think only the thin and the young are perfect and valid; being anything else is somehow shameful. We have lost sight of hundreds and hundreds of generations of other values, and we have swallowed whole what the advertising world has served up. As a result, we have sabotaged ourselves by believing that we have to be thin and we have to be perfect.

By not being thin, I could believe that the only thing wrong with me was my weight. If I dropped the pounds, I would have to face the reality that I wasn't perfect after all, or I would have to actually *be* perfect.

When I understood that rationalization, I laughed out loud. In my heart of hearts I knew I wasn't perfect and I never could be. My weight had nothing to do with my quality: it was just some extra pounds.

My weight had nothing to do with my quality: it was just some extra pounds.

While I was shedding the other perfectionistic hang-ups, I was also learning to listen to my body signals. I saw that perfect had nothing to do with me or my body. Respecting my body, caring for my body, was the issue. It was my unique temple.

As I listened to and respected my body for what it was, it began to change—almost without my noticing. I didn't eat more than was comfortable. I no longer ate for the feelings of imperfection, and the pounds began to melt off. My body wasn't becoming perfect; it was becoming what it was meant to be at its most healthy state. And if that wasn't bonus enough, I felt more at home and more at one with my body—gift upon gift—all for accepting and honoring my body for itself.

My body wasn't becoming perfect; it was becoming what it was meant to be at its most healthy state.

———————— □ ————————

Your story might be different from mine; perfectionists come in all sizes and stripes. However, if you're a perfectionist, you travel a road of tight self-control, too. To some degree, you need to conquer and manage every situation that you are in; you may have a rigid personality; you may have extraordinarily high standards of justice, fair play, and duty. You may feel that everyone should have such standards. You may feel that you know what is right, and you try your best to make everything right. You may push people away from you but feel lonely and occasionally depressed.

If you're a perfectionist, you travel a road of tight self-control.

In *Hope for the Perfectionist* Dr. David Stoop observes,

Perfectionists will work just as hard at keeping others from knowing them, as they will at changing others; they will often retreat, raising their walls and pulling up the drawbridge. They are afraid of being found wanting in some way.[1]

If you're a perfectionist, you may leave no place for *maybe* or *possibly* because your life is based on absolutes—good or bad.

- When you can't accomplish your too-high goals, you eat.
- When things don't go right, you eat.
- When people don't do what they should, you eat.
- When events don't run smoothly, you eat.
- When people don't like your behavior, you eat.

In short, you eat because the world doesn't operate the way it would if it were perfect.

In addition you may

- minimize your successes.
- maximize your failures.
- see only problems ahead.
- blame others (project) when you fall short.

Perfectionism is a particular way in which you're hard on yourself . . . organization, schedules, relationships, spirituality, or home.

Perfectionists usually have particular areas or ways in which they believe they must be perfect. Please don't think of this as your failing. *It is not a failing.* It is a particular way in which you're hard on yourself. Your area may be organization, schedules, relationships, spirituality, or home.

Because you're hard on yourself in this way, you won't allow yourself the joy of being you—until everything is just right. You're not kind to yourself, and you don't give yourself credit for doing your best. You don't forgive yourself for being human and, therefore, flawed.

It's easy to lose your way while always looking up toward one high ideal after another.

Perhaps you reached the path of perfectionism by going down the path of achievement and excellence. They aren't quite the same paths, but they're very near each other. It's easy to lose your way while always looking up toward one high ideal after another. Suddenly, you're on a strange path with a lot of stones and roots that make you stumble and bruise yourself. It's not a comfortable path.

Her pursuit of excellence became obsessive.

Laura wasn't satisfied to do just a good job; she wanted to be best. Her pursuit of excellence became obsessive, and she focused on winning her tennis matches and getting thin.

To her friends and family, Laura seemed to be doing wonderfully—at first anyway. She did better than anyone else at everything she tried, including getting top academic grades, and everyone acknowledged her as the school's best all-around female athlete. In relationships, Laura got along well with her family, and she had several close friends and a dependable boyfriend. She was also thin and attractive.

Laura had it all, or so her friends often told her. But eventually that wasn't enough. Laura wanted more—to win more, to do better in school, and to get thinner. She thought that would bring her happiness.

By her senior year, Laura's friends and parents had watched a cheerful, outgoing girl transform herself into a rigid, driven personality. They worried about her gaunt appearance and her serious, humorless view of life. No one seemed to realize that Laura was also worried about herself. "My life is falling apart," she finally told her boyfriend, "and I don't know what to do."

Laura wanted to be happy with herself as she was. But she didn't know how to get off the path of perfectionism and back on the path of achievement. No accomplishment was enough, and nothing could make her happy. (See 8-A.)

She found help and began turning her life around.

Laura wanted more—to win more, to do better in school, and to get thinner.

No accomplishment was enough.

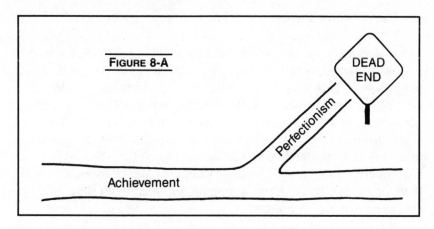

The difference between the words of a healthy achiever and a perfectionist may be:

ACHIEVEMENT	PERFECTION
"My best counts."	"Only perfect counts."
"I want to succeed."	"I'm afraid to fail."
"It's possible for me to do it."	"I settle for nothing less than perfection."
"I can choose to do my best. I can choose not to do my best."	"I must be better than anyone else."
"I want . . . I'd like . . . I wish . . ."	"I should . . . I ought . . . I must . . ."
"I want quality."	"I demand perfection."

"Anything can be viewed through the lens of moral judgment."

Family therapists Merle Fossum and Marilyn Mason wrote an insightful book called *Facing Shame*. Here's what they say about the perfectionistic family:

> Within this system of perfectionism, there may be great stress placed on control and doing things right. People are very anxious within the system, as they live under the control and demand to be right and to do right. The motto within the system may be "Anything worth doing is worth doing right," or "If I want something done right I have to do it myself," or "I can't do it well enough so I won't try." Anything can be viewed through the lens of moral judgment. Eating, cleaning, school grades, personal grooming, having money and how it is used, even physical health and mental health are subject to moral monitoring on this perfectionistic standard.[2]

"The child . . . often internalizes the goals of the parents and becomes a taskmaster."

Dr. David Stoop says,

> Parental worship of success deprives the child of personal needs, especially the need for self-direction. The child takes on the goals of the parents, which are usually impossibly perfectionistic. In addition, the child's goals are derived from the parents' own frustrations and have nothing to do with the child's interest or abilities. But the child . . . often internalizes the goals of the parents and becomes a taskmaster. . . . perfectionism can be fostered within the family by a spirit of criticism, through the observation of parents' expectations of themselves, and through the setting of extremely high standards by the parents or significant others.[3]

Briefly, here's how the perfectionistic personality comes into being. In childhood each of us begins to develop an image—an idea or concept—of the self we would like to be or think we ought to become. Some call this the ideal self. This image/ideal comes primarily from our tendency to emulate those we admire, such as our parents, relatives, teachers, peers, or characters on TV. This ego ideal exerts a potent force in determining our behavior and lifestyle.

Although all of us have some of this idealized self in us, you may be one for whom the line between the real you and the ideal self blurs. Your idealized self, some would call it the false self, could do anything or everything perfectly. As you grew older, this blurred image became what you perceived as your real self. Without your being aware of what was happening, your ideal self became your defense against failure, rejection, discouragement, and especially anxiety.

In discussing the ideal self versus the real self, Dr. Henry Cloud writes,

> Within all of us is some realization of the difference between the ideal self (the imagined perfection) and the real self (the one that truly is). If these are in a battle, we cannot function very well without conflict. We tend to be at war between what we wish were true, and what really is true. This sets up a conflict between the real and the ideal that hinders functioning.[4]

As a perfectionist, when things in your life aren't perfect, you need something that protects you from facing your real, or core, self. You direct your energy toward developing your ideal self so that you actually become flawless.

Although most people come to realize that there are few absolute standards, this is the way of life for you as a perfectionist. (See 8-B.)

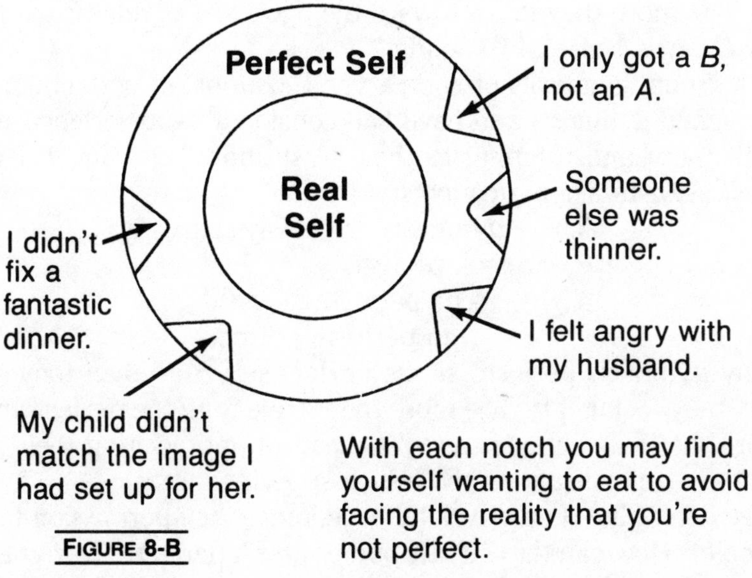

"We tend to be at war between what we wish were true, and what really is true."

Perfect Self

Real Self

I only got a *B*, not an *A*.

Someone else was thinner.

I didn't fix a fantastic dinner.

I felt angry with my husband.

My child didn't match the image I had set up for her.

With each notch you may find yourself wanting to eat to avoid facing the reality that you're not perfect.

FIGURE 8-B

That is why *should* is such an integral word in your vocabulary.

If you are a perfectionist, you

- *should* be the perfect child (or parent).
- *should* be the perfect spouse.
- *should* be the perfect friend.
- *should* be strong, able to withstand anything.
- *should* be above hurt, pain, and rejection.
- *should* have the perfect body and be the perfect weight.

NOTE TO MYSELF

Should is a four-letter word.

Unfortunately, if you get locked into thinking of yourself as this ideal self, you lose touch with your real self. This doesn't mean you're mentally unbalanced; it does mean you have no vital contact with and understanding of your real self.

I see this tendency illustrated in the way people respond to their bodies. The more they move toward the ego ideal as reality, the more they lose a true sense of the body.

As a group, gymnasts provide a vivid example of perfectionism. I have coached gymnasts and have had considerable experience working with them and listening to their frustrations. Of course, I don't mean *all* of them are perfectionists.

These gymnasts are always striving

to look perfect.

to be perfect.

to perform perfectly.

The more they strive to fit the perfect image, the more the real self fades away.

Many gymnasts perform as the perfect self. Yet when they leave the mat, they feel empty. The more they strive to fit the perfect image, the more the real self fades away. Instead of appreciating their good points, they concentrate on the less-than-perfect areas.

They don't give themselves the freedom or self-permission to like their bodies. How can they? Their bodies aren't perfect. Their goal is a flawless score with a flawless body.

When gymnasts get compulsive about perfection, they transfer the obsession to their eating and become afraid to eat. Their eating becomes erratic, and they lose sight of what their bodies really look like. At the same time, when others look at them, their eyes fill with admiration and their voices with praise. "Perfect! Wonderful!" they say. The objects of the praise say to themselves, *If only they really knew.* They are harder on themselves than anyone else is.

The gymnasts I coached said:

Their eating becomes erratic, and they lose sight of what their bodies really look like.

- "If I felt positive about myself, I might lose my motivation to work hard."
- "If I started to like my body, I might stop trying so hard, and then I'd get fat."
- "If I didn't punish myself, I might enjoy myself."
- "If I started to enjoy myself I might keep on eating and not stop."

While working with these gymnasts, I taught them to separate eating from achieving perfect, thin bodies. I wanted them to know how to eliminate self-judgment, to enjoy eating, and to accept their bodies.

I wanted them to know how to eliminate self-judgment.

Early on, I learned it didn't do any good to say, "You're too hard on yourself. Don't judge yourself anymore." That's about effective as saying, "Don't think about pink elephants."

I wanted them to learn to *own* their bodies. And in learning to own their eating and their bodies, they could begin to accept themselves. As they began to accept themselves, they could look at themselves realistically, each as an individual, not as a group trying to reach the elusive perfect image.

Lewis Bales, a highly respected dancer and choreographer, said,

Seventy-five percent of the students who come to me with prior training know only how to do steps. They know nothing about the body or energy or breathing; they know only mechanics and virtuosity.[5]

————————— ▢ —————————

I've had two verses quoted at me: "Therefore you shall be perfect, just as your Father in heaven is perfect" (Matthew 5:48 NKJV); "You shall be blameless [or 'perfect' in some translations] before the LORD your God" (Deuteronomy 18:13).

Scholars say that the word translated "perfect" actually means "brought to completion, full grown, mature." These are injunctions to obedience, not perfection; they are not demands for flawlessness. If they were, we'd read nothing in the Bible about forgiveness.

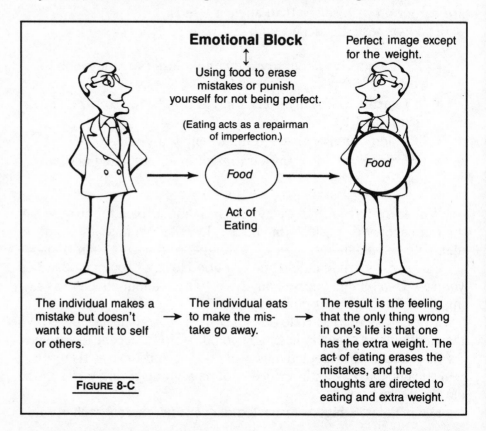

FIGURE 8-C

This is a significant problem, I've noticed, for some people who talk about God's grace and love, yet don't apply those words to themselves. Instead of receiving God's acceptance, they work harder to be perfect. Since their efforts don't bring perfection, they get depressed and feel guilty. That leads to lower self-esteem, or self-image, and often food bingeing. The inrush of food covers up the self-accusing voice—for a while.

By not being thin, you can still believe that the only thing wrong with you is your weight. You're perfect inside; you're just padded by extra food. If you drop the pounds, however, you will have to face the realization that you may not be perfect, even in areas you might have thought you were. You may have eaten to cover your feelings of imperfection and transferred your frustrations to your weight. (See 8-C.)

Facing reality is tough. It may be so difficult that you'd rather not take the steps forward. Yet I hope you will. To face the real self is scary, but it's freeing to feel like a whole person and live without constantly trying to "fix" yourself. Accepting yourself as you are now enables you to like where you are right now—at this stage of your life—your present body size and shape.

┌─ **NOTE TO MYSELF** ──────────────┐
│ *Success is the quality of the journey. Healthy eating* │
│ *emphasizes quality.* │
└────────────────────────────────────┘

When you make your own choices, you work with your real self.

When you ask yourself what you want, you get down to the core of who you are. At first you may have no idea what you really want, but stay with it. In time, you'll gain confidence in your instincts.

Accept yourself where you are. Start there. Let your real self come into focus. As this happens, the illusion of your ideal self fades.

If you feel frustrated, you may ask me

- "How many circles are *right?*"
- "How *big* should the circles be?"
- "How many fat grams should I have each day?"
- "What should I eat for breakfast?"

In response, I'll ask you,

- "What does your stomach feel like?"
- "Do you feel energized by your food?"
- "How full do you feel?"
- "Have you created a beginning and an end for each eating occasion?"

When you ask yourself what you want, you get down to the core of who you are.

- ▪ "What do you love to eat?"
- ▪ "Is eating your only pleasurable experience?"
- ▪ "What other activities do you love to do?"

———————————— □ ————————————

Your choice.   No matter what questions you may have, they come down to choice. Your choice. You choose what is right and best for you.

CHAPTER SUMMARY

Perfectionism immobilizes people and affects one's feelings and behavior. Cultural thin image promotes perfectionism. Shedding perfectionism helps people stop eating for feelings of imperfection. Perfectionists live with tight control, high expectations, and absolutes. Perfectionism is not a failing but a trap. Perfectionists are controlled and anxious (Fossum and Mason). Achieving parents can foster perfectionistic children (Stoop). The real or core self gets lost. The conflict between the real self and the ideal self hinders functioning (Cloud). *Should* denotes an impossible ideal standard. For example, gymnasts get caught up in the perfect body-score trap. They are taught to separate body from eating and accept themselves as individuals. Making choices reveals the core self. Start where you are.

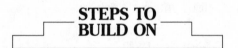

STEPS TO BUILD ON

1. Identify if and how perfectionism works in your life. How does it immobilize you? How does it limit you? How does it affect your relationships?

2. Identify if and how perfectionism affects the beginning of your eating circles and when you choose to eat.

NOTES

1. David Stoop, *Hope for the Perfectionist* (Nashville: Oliver-Nelson Books, 1989), p. 95.

2. Merle A. Fossum and Marilyn J. Mason, *Facing Shame: Families in Recovery* (New York: W. W. Norton and Company, 1986), p. 26.

3. Stoop, *Hope for the Perfectionist,* pp. 75–76.

4. Henry Cloud, *When Your World Makes No Sense* (Nashville: Oliver-Nelson Books, 1990), p. 188.

5. Philip Friedman and Gail Eisen, *The Pilates Method of Physical and Mental Conditioning* (New York: Warner Books, 1980), p. 2.

Emotions

9

Feeling Your Food?

Likely you've heard these statements or similar ones. All of them involve reward or punishment—the verbal rebuke about leaving food is a form of punishment. Each comes from a situation that carries emotional baggage.

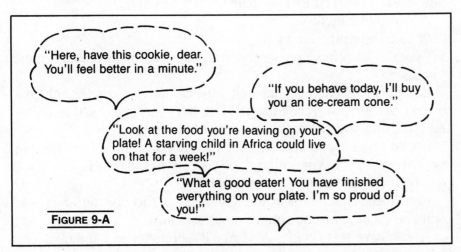

"Here, have this cookie, dear. You'll feel better in a minute."

"If you behave today, I'll buy you an ice-cream cone."

"Look at the food you're leaving on your plate! A starving child in Africa could live on that for a week!"

"What a good eater! You have finished everything on your plate. I'm so proud of you!"

FIGURE 9-A

From infancy onward, you learned to associate feelings and circumstances with food. When you cried as a baby, first you were checked to see if you were sick or wet, then, barring that, they put something into your mouth. You may have grown up in a home where food served many purposes other than nurturing your body.

For example, in some families, members consciously or unconsciously use food to

- ▪ soothe and comfort.
- ▪ reward.
- ▪ punish.
- ▪ induce guilt.
- ▪ cure emotional hurts (such as loneliness).
- ▪ hide behind (hide real selves).
- ▪ encourage overeating.

After cleaning up everything else on her plate, Dolly ate the escarole. . . . "I hate the stuff," she said.

Think about how food operated in the following situation. A woman named Dolly attended a businesswomen's banquet. The chef had garnished a lovely plate with a large leaf of escarole. After cleaning up everything else on her plate, Dolly ate the escarole.

"Why?" I asked.

"Escarole contains high levels of nutrients such as iron," and she listed the nutritional values. "And besides, I was taught to clean my plate at each meal so that we didn't waste any food."

"Do you like escarole?"

"I hate the stuff," she said.

Consider her emotions: resentment, guilt, annoyance, and a sense of invasion.

Emotional reactions connected with eating can create problems, but you can learn to recognize the link between emotional reactions and food, and you can also overcome or neutralize them.

You can change your thinking and your feelings.

It won't be easy to cut the emotional ties with food because they may have existed in your mind since your earliest days. However, you can change your thinking *and your feelings.*

Reread the statements at the beginning of this chapter. (See 9-A.) Each carries at least one serious emotional link.

"Here, have this cookie, dear. You'll feel better in a minute." *This statement imposes an emotion and tells you how to feel.*

"If you behave today, I'll buy you an ice-cream cone." *This is bribery; offering food as a reward for good behavior connects food and behavior.*

"Look at the food you're leaving on your plate! A starving child in

Africa could live on that for a week!" *You are expected to react emotionally—with guilt—to an event over which you have no control.*

"What a good eater! You have finished everything on your plate. I'm so proud of you!" *The comments encourage you to overeat and connect eating with achievement* (see chapter 7).

By now you may have thought of several other emotional ties to your eating, and you can see the close link between them. Linking food and your emotional reactions to circumstances really has nothing to do with eating to satisfy hunger and enjoying the food and your renewed energy.

It works this way:

A situation ->
    creates emotional reaction - - - - - - - - - - - - - ->
     linked with eating - - - - - - - - - - - - - - - - - - ->
      leads to emotion-eating bond.

Or here is another way of seeing this:

Something happened to you - - - - - - - - - - - - - ->
    you felt sad ->
     eating made you feel better - - - - - - - - - - - - ->
      now you feel bad because you overate!

Eventually the link operates like this:

The sight of food ->
    triggers your eating ->
     because you want to feel better.

The link between eating for energy and enjoyment and eating as an emotional reaction is individual. You may have emotional attachments to certain foods, or all foods. In fact, most of us have some of this. (See 9-B.)

Of course, you may *not* have emotional attachments to food. Your excess weight may have been the result of a lack of knowledge of the human body and how it functions or ignorance of nutritional information. If so, start listening to hunger, learning good nutritional practices, and respecting your taste buds.

Many of us still carry the messages that cause problems and tie our emotions to eating. Inner Eating will help these emotions to surface.

Start listening to hunger, learning good nutritional practices, and respecting your taste buds.

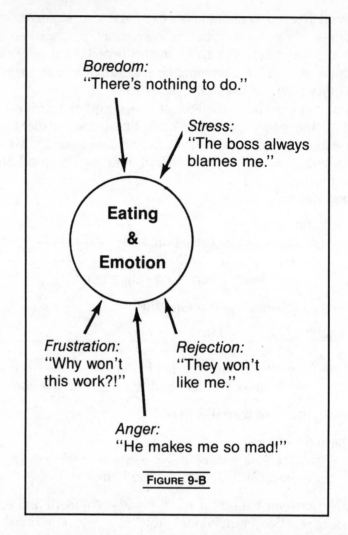

FIGURE 9-B

For example, if you get overly hungry and also hit a stressful situation, there's just too much power mounted against you, and you feel compelled to overeat. Suppose, however, that you have learned to eat only when your body requires nourishment. Then when emotions surface, you won't have two forces strengthening each other.

You first need to learn to respond to hunger signals and not emotion signals.

To become aware of your emotional reactions, you first need to learn to respond to hunger signals and not emotion signals. Then the emotion-eating link won't be so powerful, and you'll be able to separate them. You need to see that eating is eating, no matter *why* you're eating.

Your body responds to your emotions. Your body also feels hunger. To identify and separate the two feelings is the key to a successful awareness of your total self. Then you can decide which behaviors you want to keep, change, or lose. It's your choice.

Stress

For example, you can have physical reactions to stress, such as headaches or back or joint pain. Jill Dyer thought she only felt her stress in her stomach. When she felt the stress, she ate. However, after she identified hunger and stress, and fed only her hunger, she discovered that she also felt stress in her neck, which was causing upper back problems. Once she became aware of her stress, she could do exercises that would relax her. As a result, she began to lose weight and reduce her neck stress—which alleviated her back problems. By separating eating from stress, she solved two problems: (1) back and neck aches and (2) overweight.

Anger

You have a powerful emotion surging inside, such as anger. You can't ignore your feeling, so you have to do something with it. You eat, like some people smoke or drink, or you get angry with others.

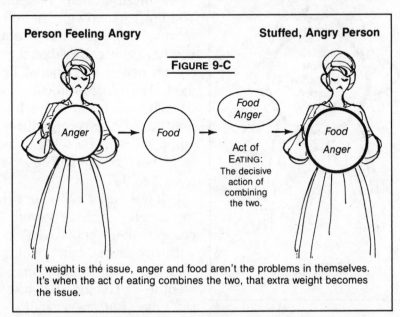

Person Feeling Angry   **Stuffed, Angry Person**

FIGURE 9-C

Anger → Food →

Food Anger

Act of
EATING:
The decisive
action of
combining
the two.

→ Food Anger

If weight is the issue, anger and food aren't the problems in themselves. It's when the act of eating combines the two, that extra weight becomes the issue.

Suppose you're angry with your employer or your neighbor or your spouse, and you feel powerless—although you may not be—so you turn to food. (See 9-C.) Yet it's more than just turning to food. It's more like an irresistible magnet.

You eat. The problem doesn't go away, but food stuffs the emotion down. That is, you cover the anger with the food. As you eat, you calm down. In a matter of minutes, the emotion feels smaller, less intense, even though the problem hasn't changed. It's the food equivalent of counting to a hundred.

Because your food intake has softened your emotion, you can now look again at the circumstances. You may still be angry but not with the same intensity. Or you could say that you exchanged the problem. You're less intense but at what price? You traded intensity for calories. You bundle up the emotion and stuff it inside your body. If you continue this style of coping with anger, you already know the result—added girth and pounds.

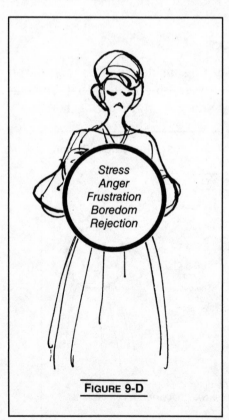

FIGURE 9-D

To make the situation worse, you focus on the secondary issue, your weight, and ignore the more important one, dealing with your anger. The weight issue becomes more intense than your anger. You don't experience the release from solving your anger because you have concentrated on the secondary matter and ignored, or denied, the primary difficulty.

With each unresolved emotion that you covered with food, you protected yourself and didn't learn how to deal with that emotion. (See 9-D.)

"It was easier and safer to face my weight," said one person, "because I didn't know what to do with my anger. I kept thinking that a diet would cure my weight—if I could find just the right diet. But I never did."

Rejection

Rejection is a feeling that comes in an infinite number of sizes from a small dart to a killer cannon. If you eat your feelings, something as small as being criticized or as large as being divorced or fired from a job can trigger your eating. Some people store the memory of old hurts so that even a small rejection is magnified out of proportion. If you use food for comfort and reassurance, you may eat to reduce the overpowering feelings of rejection. (See 9-E.) Therefore, if you identify the eating you do to ease feelings of rejection and then separate that from eating to ease feelings of hunger, you empower yourself to stop the eating you don't want or need.

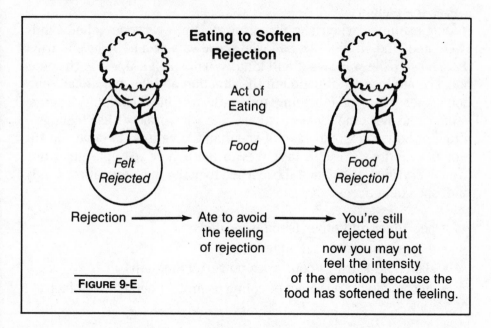

Eating to Soften Rejection

Act of Eating

Food

Felt Rejected

Food Rejection

Rejection ⟶ Ate to avoid the feeling of rejection ⟶ You're still rejected but now you may not feel the intensity of the emotion because the food has softened the feeling.

FIGURE 9-E

Frustration

Another client said, "Eating a lot of food made it easier for me to handle problems. I could sail through life in spite of any difficulties, and I honestly believed that I handled everything well. My only problem was my extra weight. I was dealing with everything well and complimented myself for being so even-keeled. Yet every day I'd think, *If only my weight was where I want it, everything would be perfect.*" So she resolved to diet. She had missed the primary problem by focusing on the secondary problem. (See 9-F.)

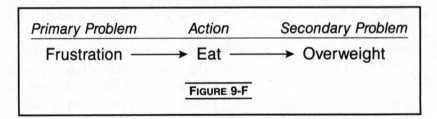

Primary Problem	Action	Secondary Problem
Frustration ⟶	Eat ⟶	Overweight

FIGURE 9-F

Dieting is a predictable and usually unsuccessful way to cope with the issue of weight. It *is* unsuccessful because it doesn't confront what causes the weight.

For example, when she was growing up, everyone called Cindy sweet and kind. In time she believed she always had to behave in ways that showed she was sweet and kind. When she felt upset with someone, she ate instead of handling the situation and her emotional reaction. After years of following this pattern, Cindy couldn't separate eating from her emotional reactions. She was afraid of her feelings— afraid of how she would react if she didn't have food to cover up the human emotions. Cindy's task was to learn how to separate eating from everything else. Once she learned to make that separation, Cindy said, she could accept that

She was afraid of her feelings—afraid of how she would react if she didn't have food to cover up the human emotions.

- her anger and other feelings existed.
- it was normal to feel anger.
- she could learn to cope with powerful emotions.
- she couldn't use the act of eating to protect herself from feelings.

┌─**NOTE TO MYSELF**─────────────────┐
My body feels the impact of my emotions, for which I am responsible.
└────────────────────────────────────┘

The Inner Eating process will help you accomplish the reunion of your thinking, feeling, and physical selves into a whole and self-respecting person.

Throughout this book I refer to holding (or making) your body responsible. People with weight and/or emotional problems often feel disconnected from their bodies, as though their minds and bodies are not a single, interdependent unit. If you feel this disconnection, perhaps seeing yourself only from the neck up, perhaps referring to your body as "it" instead of "me," you are implying that your body is responsible for itself, that what goes in your head has nothing to do with it. Not true. The Inner Eating process will help you accomplish the reunion of your thinking, feeling, and physical selves into a whole and self-respecting person.

When you overeat, your body gains weight. If you can honestly think in terms of "I gained weight because . . . ," you are holding yourself responsible for the treatment of your body.

Dr. Henry Cloud says it this way:

> I am responsible for taking care of my body. I must "guard it." . . . I best know what it requires to get needs met. For example, I feel my hunger, and I take responsibility for knowing that and for doing something about it. If I feel pain, I am responsible for telling someone about the pain who has knowledge to help it. That responsibility is mine even if I did not inflict the pain, for it is my pain, it is in my body. Since it is in my body, I must own it and be responsible for it.[1]

Once you separate your eating for emotional reasons from eating for nourishment, and you eat only to take care of your body, your emotions will have a chance to surface. These deeply hidden feelings are yours. They're inside you. Own them. (See 9-G.)

Because it's so important for you to see these as two distinct issues, I'll state them again.

1. Eating is for caring for your physical needs.

2. When you separate that from eating for emotional reasons, you allow your stuffed-inside emotions to surface and be recognized so that you can feel them and learn to cope with them.

Having a weight problem doesn't mean you lack willpower because the power of your determination isn't the issue. Using willpower actually means you are working against your body. It's as if you are saying, "Body, you don't know what's going on, but my head does." The mind and the body are separate parts of the same organism, communicating through the control panel of the brain. Body communication is, technically speaking, chemical reactions to specific needs. So, if your body requires food or rest, or oxygen or a temperature change, it

Using willpower actually means you are working against your body.

If you're uncomfortable physically from being hungry or stuffed, and emotionally from unresolved problems, you may be trying to solve both by eating inappropriately.

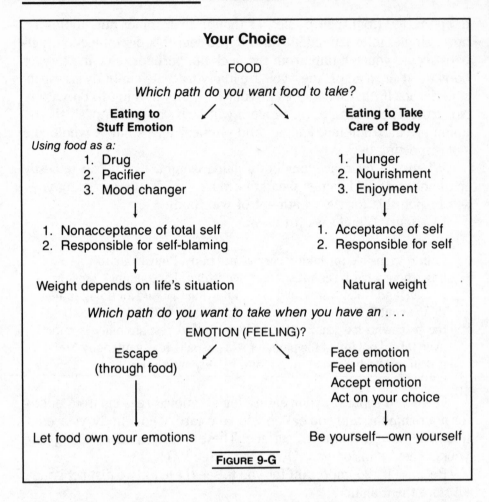

Your Choice

FOOD

Which path do you want food to take?

**Eating to   Eating to Take
Stuff Emotion   Care of Body**

Using food as a:

1. Drug	1. Hunger
2. Pacifier	2. Nourishment
3. Mood changer	3. Enjoyment

1. Nonacceptance of total self	1. Acceptance of self
2. Responsible for self-blaming	2. Responsible for self

Weight depends on life's situation   Natural weight

Which path do you want to take when you have an . . .

EMOTION (FEELING)?

Escape   Face emotion
(through food)   Feel emotion
          Accept emotion
          Act on your choice

Let food own your emotions   Be yourself—own yourself

FIGURE 9-G

calls for it in the appropriate way. You'll feel the need to eat, sleep, breathe deeply, or put on or take off a sweater. If you don't listen to your body's signals, you can expect to get increasingly uncomfortable. If you're uncomfortable physically from being hungry or stuffed, and emotionally from unresolved problems, you may be trying to solve both by eating inappropriately. By struggling, withholding food, and putting yourself on restrictive diets, you make life more difficult for yourself. If you separate the two issues (emotions and body care), you can learn to handle both better.

Here are five steps to help you.

1. Ask yourself what you're feeling or what may have happened that triggered your urge to eat. (You have already learned how to as-

Ask yourself what you're feeling or what may have happened that triggered your urge to eat.

sess your hunger when you start and stop eating—the numbers to the left and right of your eating circle—so you will recognize when you're about to eat for a nonhunger reason [i.e., when you're at a 6 and still reach for food.]) *Recognizing and accepting your emotional entanglement in eating* is a major breakthrough.

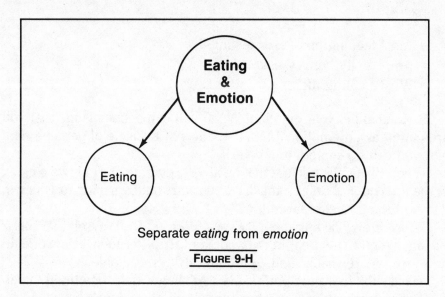

Separate *eating* from *emotion*

FIGURE 9-H

For example, a young devout Christian who is filled with inner rage has never been able to express his feelings openly. His father is also a devout Christian and constantly reminds him that "good Christians" just don't get angry. If you watch him eat, he actually *attacks* his food. The more angry he feels, the greater the amount he consumes and the more numerous his eating circles.

Or there's Jeff, who ate when he got bored. Afterward he felt disgusted with himself for eating when he wasn't hungry. He said, "I hated that overstuffed feeling, and I loathed myself for being so weak-willed."

2. Disconnect the emotion from eating. Because you have linked the two together for so long, they operate like Siamese twins. As soon as you feel the emotion, even on a subconscious level, it acts like a magnet that draws you to food. This same dynamic operates in people who use tobacco or alcohol to medicate emotions.

Sometimes the cause becomes obvious, such as the yearning to eat immediately after your boss or coworker has rebuffed you. Or you feel

Disconnect the emotion from eating.

inadequate to make a speech. Or you're worried about something. These discoveries tend to come about more easily when you're keeping a daily journal.

You can break this powerful attraction by eating smaller amounts of food each time. As you eat, think about what you are feeling. Ask yourself,

- Am I feeding hunger or feelings?
- Am I really hungry now?
- What's eating me?

Acknowledge that you are eating as an emotional reaction.

3. Rechannel your emotion. When you can acknowledge that you are eating as an emotional reaction and not because of genuine hunger, you can do something about it.

When Bill Quick told me that he always overate around two o'clock in the afternoon, I asked him, "Did you start out by saying to yourself, 'I'm not going to overeat today'?"

"Absolutely," he answered. "Every morning I tell myself that this is the day when I won't eat in the middle of the afternoon." He works in an office where snacks and coffee are always available.

"That's the first problem," I said. "Allow yourself something to eat. Just make sure you create a beginning and an ending."

"Okay, I'll try that," he said.

"What else could you do after you finish a circle of eating?" I asked him.

He couldn't think of a thing.

He had a variety of choices and continuing to eat until he was stuffed was only one option.

"Think about it some more. Give me six things you could do after you've eaten." I wanted him to realize that he had a variety of choices and that continuing to eat until he was stuffed was only one option. Bill had gotten into the habit of eating when he didn't have work pressuring him. He was feeding the space of open time. He started out "a little hungry" and then kept on eating.

"I could walk around the block," he said.

"Would you do that?" I asked.

He shook his head.

"I don't want to count that then. Tell me six things you could do and would do."

Agonizingly, he realized that eating was the only thing he thought about when he had open time. So he worked at creating options for his free moments. "I could arrange to return telephone calls during that period."

"Very good," I said. "You have five more to go."

It took Bill several minutes, but he finally came up with six things to substitute. The idea was to shift the emotion away from eating when he had open time. By isolating the factor of open time from the act of eating, he could begin to cut down on the amounts and frequency of his snacking. Before long, Bill recognized his open time easily and dealt with it appropriately instead of with food.

Focus on the emotion behind the eating. Food can hide, cover up, or mask the problems of your inner life. Even after nibbling or gorging yourself, you're still left with the basic emotional problem.

Focus on the emotion behind the eating.

In my case, I've always been an achiever and quite competitive. Tennis is my favorite sport. One day I didn't play well. In fact I lost the game. When I came home from the match, without thinking, I started to eat. I was hungry, or so I thought. Yet as I reached for the food, I paused to ask myself, Why am I doing this? Am I really hungry?

As I reflected, I realized that being hungry had nothing to do with my reaching for food. I felt annoyed, disappointed, hurt, and even a little self-rejected for not playing well. Because I hadn't acknowledged the powerful reaction to losing a tennis match, my most obvious way to numb my feeling was through my stomach.

When I had acknowledged what I felt, and where it came from, I didn't feel the need to eat. I had acknowledged the major issue of my feelings about the tennis match instead of eating to stuff down my hurt and disappointment.

No matter what you're feeling, you can identify it and probably the source. Then you can find ways that don't involve food to deal with those emotions. Keeping a journal is a helpful tool during such times. Writing out your feelings enables you to concentrate on the emotion, its cause, and what to do about it.

Writing out your feelings enables you to concentrate on the emotion, its cause, and what to do about it.

Sometimes you can't isolate a particular cause. It may be too deep-seated to deal with alone. Or even if you know the cause, perhaps it's too big or too painful to struggle with by yourself. If this is true for you, please don't hesitate to seek professional help.

There is a gift we give ourselves when we separate emotions and eating: energy. While we blunt the sharp edge of emotion with food,

Make choices.

we also blunt the buoyancy of energy. Once we free ourselves of the oppression of food, we find renewed enthusiasm, stamina, and even joy.

4. Enjoy your eating. After you have discovered the role emotions play in your eating, you will realize you can make choices. You have the power within to change your eating pattern. You can choose whether to eat or not, depending on your hunger level.

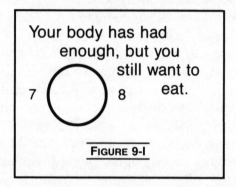

FIGURE 9-I

CHAPTER SUMMARY

Feelings and food are tied to eating problems. The emotion of emptiness feels like hunger, which you mask with food. Food becomes a companion, so weight—the secondary problem—is dealt with, not the emotion—the primary problem. The combination of weight and emotional problems fosters a mind-body split. (See 9-I.) Assessing your hunger level can reveal if you're eating for emotion or hunger. Eating for an emotional reason robs your energy; facing and releasing the emotion from the bondage of food return energy.

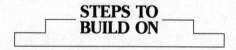

STEPS TO
BUILD ON

1. Use your circles to determine if you are eating for hunger or for an emotional reason.

2. When you find that you're eating for emotional reasons, consider other options at the moment. Try to list six other options for eating.

3. Use your journal to explore roots of the emotion(s) behind emotion-based eating.

4. Prepare to discover new energy and enthusiasm.

<u>NOTE</u>

1. Henry Cloud, *When Your World Makes No Sense* (Nashville: Oliver-Nelson Books, 1990), p. 107.

10

Voices Within

Do you recognize the chatter that goes on inside your head? Some of the things you hear may be:

"I hate liver and onions, but they're good for me."

"I hate to prepare the food."

"If only I didn't have this addiction to chocolate."

"I'll eat this and then skip dinner."

"There's always tomorrow to start my diet."

"Why did I keep eating?"

"I'm going to eat it! So there!"

"I've got those thin clothes in my closet. Will I ever wear them again?"

"I'm tired of depriving myself."

"Since I can't do anything about my eating, I might as well admit that I'm going to be fat."

"If only I could lose ten pounds."

"I can't waste this good food."

"Why did I eat that?"

"Oh, well, I've blown it; I'll keep eating."

"Mmmm, that smells so good."

"I'll just have a taste."

"My hostess will feel bad if I refuse."

"Why did he give me so much to eat?"

"How does he stay so thin?"

"If I eat this candy, I'll develop fat hips like my mother."

"What am I going to eat?"

"I'll exercise more tomorrow."

"Just one potato chip can't do much harm."

"I've been good all week."

"Look at the amount he eats. If I ate that much . . ."

"There's nothing I can do about my weight anyway."

"Why couldn't I be born with a stiletto figure?"

"How does he stay so thin?"

"Just as soon as this diet's over, I'm going to . . ."

"I'm digging my grave with my teeth."

"If I could just have somebody prepare my meals, I wouldn't have a problem with weight."

"How could anyone love a person like me?"

"If my wife wasn't always on my case, I could be thin."

"Why are my clothes so tight? Now I've got to buy something that fits."

"If I eat it, I'll get fat."

"I'd like myself a lot more if I were just twenty pounds lighter."

"If I tried harder, I know I could stay on a diet."

"I feel like a fat, overstuffed cow."

These inner voices influence our eating.

I've known only two people who had no chatter about food going round and round in their heads. For the rest of us, these inner voices influence our eating as much as any other problem.

That constant mental heckling steals your freedom of choice and keeps you eating for reasons other than need for nutrition. I've lived with those voices, too. Some of them were of my own making; others I inherited from my family and our culture. The more chatter you have, the faster you may eat—or with all the chatter you may fear eating. You may sense a "racing feeling" when you're around food. (See 10-A.) *Calm the chatter*—relax—slow down and ask yourself, (1) Do I like this food? (2) Am I hungry?

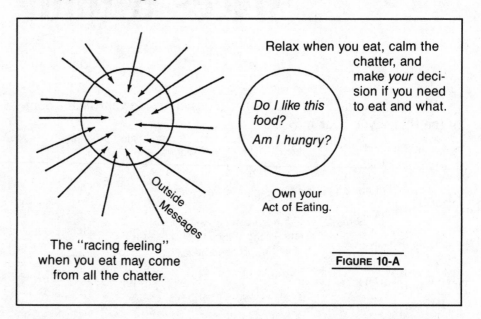

Relax when you eat, calm the chatter, and make *your* decision if you need to eat and what.

Do I like this food?

Am I hungry?

Outside Messages

Own your Act of Eating.

The "racing feeling" when you eat may come from all the chatter.

FIGURE 10-A

When I first started writing this book, I saw Dennis Anderson at a ski meeting and dinner. We talked about the chatter—messages that get attached to our eating, which "usually develop during childhood," I said.

It was a game to see if he could get extra food.

"Don't I know it!" he exclaimed. He told me that his double-barreled problem of eating a lot and never wasting food came as a result of feeling he never had enough to eat as a child. He and his brother raced home at noon, and the first one in the house got the bigger portion of food. No one ever had seconds; there was never any food left. When he was growing up, Dennis learned to adopt mothers who loved to feed him. It was a game to see if he could get extra food.

As an adult, Dennis became quite successful in his field. The amount of food available was almost limitless, but the early messages of "grab fast" were still playing in his head.

Dennis never learned how to listen to his body because those messages (referred to also as scripts or tapes) from childhood jammed his receptors. He couldn't discern his body's signals.

He couldn't discern his body's signals.

Dennis had to convince himself that he could

- hear a different voice.
- erase the old tapes.
- learn to hear his body speak to him.

Childhood head-chatter was causing him to overeat at practically every meal, and maintaining his weight had become a struggle. Once Dennis recognized the source of the messages, he could rewrite the script and begin listening to his body.

Once Dennis recognized the source of the messages, he could rewrite the script.

While Dennis and I sat at the table, he said, "Look at my plate." He had left a small amount on it. "Two years ago I would have felt that I had to go back for seconds. Then I'd feel uncomfortably stuffed the rest of the night."

"And now?" I asked.

"I'm satisfied with one helping, and that's all I need. I don't feel compelled to go back for more." He smiled. "And you know what? My body feels great when I'm finished!"

Cindy Harris also remembered her old script. She would get praise and lots of attention when she would eat a lot of food. "How can you eat that much? What a good eater you are!" She would challenge others to eating contests and usually win. As she got older, it was difficult to erase such a fun relationship with food. When she would eat small amounts the enjoyment just wasn't there until she could learn to recognize her old tapes and erase them from her act of eating.

Another man who had two brothers remembers racing to see who could eat faster and consume more quantity. With two brothers at the table, he didn't have much time to think whether he was enjoying the food. If he stopped to think about it, there would be none left! Once the old feeling of not getting any food unless he ate fast was removed, he could relax and enjoy his food in small quantities.

Chatter blankets our instinct.

We're all born with the instinct to hear and respond to the body's calls for food, and we use that instinct as infants. The chatter that eventually covers the instinct is based in our emotions and comes from sources outside ourselves. It blankets our instinct, but it doesn't kill it. It can be uncovered again.

Be aware of your chatter.

A big step for you in the Inner Eating process is learning to be aware of your chatter. Most people are so used to the inner noise that they can hardly hear the voice of their instincts anymore.

By bringing our thoughts into captivity, we are taking responsibility for them.

We must take responsibility for our thinking and the development of our minds. Many people do not think very often about what they think about. They just let their thoughts live inside the head without observing them or questioning them. In short, they don't own their thoughts. But by bringing our thoughts into captivity, we are taking responsibility for them and evaluating them, considering what they mean about the status of our hearts and minds. We are owning them.[1]

Sometimes just listening to your body will work if the chatter isn't too firmly ingrained. When I say, "Listen to your body," some clients pick up on it immediately. When I add, "Eat only when you're hungry," it works because they don't have to combat a head filled with chatter.

If you're like most people, the chatter has been in your head so long that you don't question it.

They're the rare ones. If you're like most people, the chatter has been in your head so long that you don't question it; you just obey.

Let's say that when you were growing up, money was tight, and making ends meet was a struggle. Your father might have said, "Eat up. We don't know if we'll have a full meal tomorrow."

You accepted what he said, even if you never missed a meal. As an adult the old message still says, "Better eat up. You don't know if you'll have anything to eat tomorrow." If you examine it, you'll see the old tape isn't appropriate because you know you have plenty of food available. You know you won't starve. But the message you hear is an emotional one, and it's also someone else's rule that you internalized. Until you start to question the accuracy of the voices within, you continue to obey as they dictate.

Read the messages in the diagram. You may recognize them as some of your chatter. All of them are internal messages that give you instructions. They say things such as:

- You *must* have your vegetables.
- Don't waste your food!
- Better eat now. You might not get any later.

The messages seem to intrude on everything you think and do. But you don't *have* to listen to them. You can turn them off (yes, you can!), and you can argue with them. Or even better, you can decide what kind of chatter goes on. After all, it is your mind that's involved.

You could start with this.

┌─**NOTE TO MYSELF**────────────────────────┐
│
│ *I can choose my own messages. I can write my own*
│ *messages.*
│
└──┘

Mental chatter and emotional issues are usually combined because the chatter grows out of the emotional issues. To become aware of the chatter is to become aware of the emotional issues and strengthen your ability to identify and resolve with the two. Once identified, the chatter can be rewritten and/or abolished, the emotional issues dealt with, and your eating instincts reclaimed.

To become aware of the chatter is to become aware of the emotional issues.

──────────────────── □ ────────────────────

Because you may have been using food to solve your problems—or so it seems—you need to move beyond that. One way is to think through the situation. You can reason it out with yourself.

──────────────────── □ ────────────────────

Bonnie had worked hard to separate stressful situations from food. Then she went through a difficult time because of her mother's lingering illness. Afterward she said, "I realized that I used food to help me through that stressful time."

She had made a start on the surface areas of her life, but as the stress deepened, she reached for food again. Only afterward could she see how much she relied on food as a problem solver.

Previously, after she'd realized she'd gained weight, the voices in her head would have said, "You need to go on a diet!" focusing on the food issue, not the emotional issue. Now Bonnie is aware of her inclination to eat under stress and can disconnect stress and eating, and she can change her inner voices to support her decision.

When you disconnect, start small.

Bonnie didn't resort to dieting. Instead she worked on disconnecting the chatter that mixed her eating due to stress with eating to take care of her body. When you disconnect, start small. Don't attempt to change everything immediately. As you accept this need to disconnect, become aware of the times and circumstances. A journal can be of immense help here.

Eating under stress doesn't feel good.

Once you start to disassociate eating and other issues, you'll understand your pattern. You'll recognize that eating under stress doesn't feel good. When you've disconnected under a little stress, you can handle it on bigger issues.

Handle the underlying problem first.

As you progress, you may discover that what appeared to be an easy solution—eating for instant gratification—is actually a bigger problem. You can see that you don't want to ignore the real issue, the bigger problem, to be able to concentrate on your weight. Instead, handle the underlying problem first. You really can!

By being aware that you are responding to inner chatter and old patterns, you can turn off the voices. You can feel the tensions. Once you start feeling the stress, you won't want to eat.

If you eat under stress, the body isn't equipped to handle the digestion necessary.

Stress and food don't mix. The body's natural response to stress is the fight-or-flight response; a rush of adrenaline causes the body's blood to rush to the brain and the extremities—away from the stomach. So, if you eat under stress, the body isn't equipped to handle the digestion necessary. By dealing with the issue at hand instead of trying to eat it, you'll discover that you feel less uncomfortable, in both body and mind.

You probably have another kind of chatter in your head, too. I've separated these thoughts because they are somewhat different. Most of the chatter comes from your own head. You may have picked up some of it from others and internalized it, but it's your chatter.

This second kind of inner chatter centers on three key words: *should; ought;* and *must.* The next time you hear a sentence in your head using any of these hammer words, listen closely. You need to identify them.

What are some of these messages?

- I shouldn't eat so much.
- I ought to be able to cut down.

- I should always finish everything on my plate.
- I ought to eat broccoli because it's good for me.
- I should eat what my mother has taken so many hours to prepare.
- I should be able to lose weight.
- I ought to look better in my clothes.
- I really must eat something nutritious.

For several reasons, these are the toughest inner messages you struggle with.

1. While the other messages are tentative, these are authoritarian. They command; they insist; they offer you no choice; they give you no opportunity to question. Then there are the absolutes, such as *always* and *never*.

- I must always clean my plate.
- I must never allow waste.
- I should never eat sugar.
- I should never refuse food.

2. These inner messages pile on guilt. When you hear "should," it's almost like God speaking; disobedience endangers your soul.

- You shouldn't eat that.
- If you do, you'll get fat.
- You ought to eat vegetables.
- Children in Ethiopia are starving because you throw away so much food.

No logical connection exists between people starving and your wasting food. You behave a certain way because you have been taught to behave that way.

3. You are listening to another's voice. This point is important. Those three guilt-inducing words in your head aren't your words; they belong to somebody else. If you listen carefully enough, you'll be able to identify the speaker.

Cec Murphey told me that as an adult, he wouldn't have considered going to bed without a heavy snack. By listening carefully to his yearnings for that snack, he began to distinguish the voice of his mother.

No logical connection exists between people starving and your wasting food.

Cec's parents were farmers in Oklahoma during the double trouble of the dust bowl and the Great Depression, and the family lost everything. For the rest of her life, his mother talked about having to go to bed hungry during those terrible years. He internalized that message to hear her say, "You shouldn't go to bed hungry."

The biggest problem with listening to someone else's voice is that it is someone else's. He or she has values and beliefs that are now going through your head. You don't have to live by anyone else's values; you have the right to make your own choices. You don't have to be a prisoner, held in bondage by someone else's "should," "ought," or "must."

You have the right to make your own choices.

Each time the chatter tells you what you ought to do, question the words, challenge the voice, and make your own decision. The best way I know to combat a "should tape" is to ask one question: Why?

Question the words, challenge the voice, and make your own decision.

I do this in talking with clients who have had problems with chatter in their heads. For instance, when Connie was telling me about her eating, I asked, "Do you feel you should eat everything on your plate?"

"Of course," she said, without hesitating.

"Why?"

She stared at me before she finally said, "Nobody has ever asked me that question before."

"Did anybody ever say to you that you had to finish your food?"

She thought about it and then shook her head.

"Then why do you have to finish your food?"

"I don't know. I suppose I just thought I should."

"Exactly the problem," I said. "You're listening to a voice that's not your choice."

"You're listening to a voice that's not your choice."

Or when I asked one woman the question about anybody telling her to clean her plate, she had an immediate answer.

"My dad. He wouldn't let us leave the table if he could see one speck of food."

"Is your father still around and still controlling your eating?"

"Oh, no," she said. "I haven't lived at home for twelve years."

"You mean that you left home twelve years ago, yet your father still tells you how to eat?"

"I never thought of it that way before," she said.

"Most of us have voices from the past that try to control our lives," I said. "That's all right if you agree with their messages and you want them to become your own."

"Most of us have voices from the past that try to control our lives."

Sometimes I'll ask, "Why do you feel you have to have something nutritious every time you eat?" They usually have no answer.

A quarter of a century ago, Eric Berne said that most of us are taught early in life to follow what he called scripts. He said that we are scripted (*programmed* is the more common term now) primarily by our parents—verbally and nonverbally. They teach us how to live to the best of their ability. Our parents' behaviors, attitudes, and choices shape our childhood perceptions and beliefs. Then we may live out countless "shoulds." These scripts become a guide for life—unless we do something to change them. We can erase the old tapes, or parts of them, Berne said, and make new ones for ourselves.

Your childhood days may have contained words or ideas that sounded like the following:

- "You need three big meals every day."
- "It's mealtime, so we eat."
- "Finish your food."
- "We always have a big evening meal."

What such people don't realize is that they do have options. They can make their own choices. For example, they could

- cut the number of circles in half.
- say no to eating occasionally.
- stop eating before they feel stuffed.

Some of my clients need permission not to feel stuffed because it goes contrary to the "should" feeling of childhood. When we discuss their options, they say, "Oh, I never even thought of that." Or "I assumed that's how I was supposed to feel."

Once we start talking about the inner chatter and identifying it, I usually work a grid with them. Because I don't know what's inside other people's heads, I have them draw it out so they can see that the words and choices are their own and not mine.

I usually start by saying, "Give me six reasons you thought you overate at dinner." (They may not be sure of the main reason; that's why I use a grid.) They give me six reasons, and then I start asking them which they felt was more important.

Here are Chris's responses:

1. It tasted so good.
2. It smelled so good.
3. I had to finish my food.
4. It was dinnertime.
5. Being stuffed was always the feeling of ending the evening meal when I was a child.
6. I deserved it.

I noticed that not one answer involved taking care of her body, which is not unusual.

"Chris," I said, "I want you to relax. Close your eyes. Visualize yourself at the table. You have overeaten. Concentrate on how your body feels."

Once Chris put herself back into that moment, we did the comparing grid using her six responses. (See 10-B.)

```
①— 2
①— 3     ②— 3
1 —④     2 —④     3 —④
1 —⑤     2 —⑤     3 —⑤     4 —⑤
1 —⑥     2 —⑥     3 —⑥     4 —⑥     5 —⑥
```

FIGURE 10-B

When we counted her choices, Chris's answers came out like this:

2—1. It tasted so good.
1—2. It smelled so good.
0—3. I had to finish my food.
3—4. It was dinnertime.
4—5. Being stuffed was always the feeling of ending the evening meal when I was a child.
5—6. I deserved it.

This is the same list in priority order:

1. I deserved it.
2. Being stuffed was always the feeling of ending the evening meal when I was a child.
3. It was dinnertime.
4. It tasted so good.
5. It smelled so good.
6. I had to finish my food.

Before we began, Chris thought her problem was that the food tasted so good. She could see that wasn't the real issue. The response about its smelling so good didn't have much bearing, either. Her two significant reasons for overeating were (1) she deserved it, and (2) feeling stuffed was the way she had learned to eat as a child.

Seeing her choices provided Chris with insight about her eating. She could resolve the old messages by erasing them, and she could start listening to her body. But until that moment, the old tapes playing inside her head drowned out her ability to hear her body speak.

Resolve the old messages by erasing them.

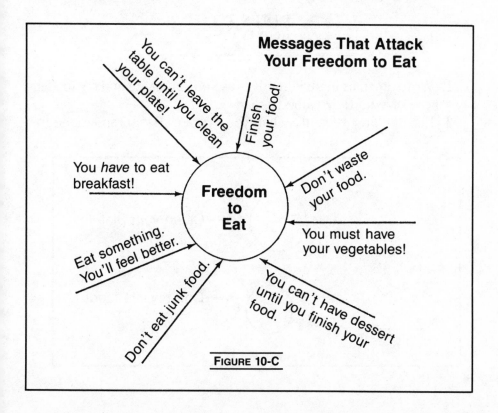

Messages That Attack Your Freedom to Eat

You can't leave the table until you clean your plate!

Finish your food!

Don't waste your food.

You *have* to eat breakfast!

Freedom to Eat

Eat something. You'll feel better.

You must have your vegetables!

Don't eat junk food.

You can't have dessert until you finish your food.

FIGURE 10-C

"When you make choices, you can silence those voices."

Just as it was with Chris, the person is usually amazed when I finish the grid. "Remember," I emphasize, "I'm not telling you why you over-eat. You discovered that for yourself. When you make choices, you can silence those voices. If I make the choices for you, I'm only adding more chatter."

CHAPTER SUMMARY

Inner chatter heckles you about your eating, urging you to eat more than you want. (See 10-C.) The chatter can be identified as directives from the past. Obeying inner voices covers your healthy instincts. Mental chatter and emotional issues can be identified and separated and dealt with. Eating when stressed, or for reasons of stress, taxes a body poised to fight or run. Guilt-inducing chatter can be identified as some other person's voice.

STEPS TO BUILD ON

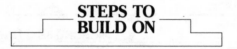

1. Write down as many directives as you can name and try to identify where or who they came from.
2. Recall a time recently when you overate. Try to remember any

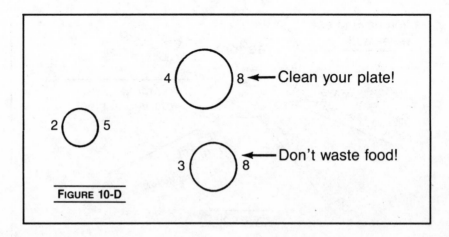

FIGURE 10-D

voices that urged you to eat beyond your balance point. Use the sample diagram (see 10-D), or journaling, as you are comfortable.

NOTE

1. Henry Cloud, *When Your World Makes No Sense* (Nashville: Oliver-Nelson Books, 1990), p. 113.

11

The Function of Boundaries

Many years ago, I read a story about Ellis Park. The woman who told it said that when she lived in a large city and was always surrounded by crowds of people, she felt crushed and yet alone. One day she found a little park hidden in the city, a little cloister of quiet and trees and birds. There she would go to renew herself and restore her inner peace. Then she had to move to another city, and she despaired of ever finding another Ellis Park.

You, too, can have a place of renewal.

To her surprise, she discovered that she carried away with her the peace and restoration of the park in a very private place near her heart. She could go to that park any time she chose and find its gift of quiet and strength. You, too, she told her readers, can have a place of renewal, an Ellis Park inside yourself, and you can make it look like and sound like anything you choose.

That story stayed with me, and I have learned to employ the concept it teaches. But it wasn't until years later that I recognized she was talking about what, in psychological circles, is called boundaries.

Boundaries aren't walls; they're choices.

Boundaries, as I said in an earlier chapter, are internal limits that we set for ourselves. They are limits for what we will and won't do, how and when we will allow other people to influence us, and what our values will be. Boundaries aren't walls; they're choices.

Internal boundaries are necessary to keep from being crushed as unique individuals.

Although the psychological discussion of boundaries is relatively recent, I believe the concept can be seen working in the human community as far back as we care to look. For example, when large numbers of people are crowded into a small area, internal boundaries are necessary to keep from being crushed as unique individuals. What better example can we find of that than the inner calm and traditional Oriental courtesy of Japanese people. I see their small traditional gardens as examples of a cultural Ellis Park, designed to impart serenity in a place where space is extraordinarily limited. I see their traditional courtesy as an example of a centuries-old practice of honoring the external and internal boundaries of others.

Families can be (and often are) places of boundary invasion, where children are not encouraged to build healthy boundaries—mostly because parents are not aware of what boundaries are, how they function, and how to build them—or where instinctive boundaries are invaded through harsh domination, emotional, physical, and/or sexual abuse. Generally, though, invasion isn't intentional, and boundary destruction is caused by ill-guided good intentions.

Since, first, the invasion was essentially benign, and second, we can't go back and relive our childhoods, the most productive move we can make now is to understand the concept of boundaries, encourage ourselves to build healthy ones, and then accept their gracious gift of spiritual strength and serenity.

A good place to start is to see how the concept works in Inner Eating. Boundaries are interior and personal; eating is a strictly personal activity done for the purpose of physical maintenance—in spite of any social conventions we have attached to it. Healthy boundaries encourage healthy eating habits without intrusion from other people.

Your boundaries have been invaded by various forces and influences from the environment, such as family, spouse, and cultural ideals and images. These invasions have given you voices and scripts that hide your choices from you. But Inner Eating helps you become aware of both the voices and the fact that you have the birthright of choice.

The process of Inner Eating returns ownership of your choices, your boundaries, to you, beginning with using the circles to define each eating occasion. That definition shows that you are in very real control of that specific boundary. You have taken it back from whoever or whatever took it from you in the first place, and it belongs to no one else.

Learning to feel your food, your hunger, and your fullness, as you did when you were a child, is a step in reclaiming your body, the tem-

Boundary destruction is caused by ill-guided good intentions.

The most productive move we can make now is to understand the concept of boundaries.

Healthy boundaries encourage healthy eating habits.

You have the birthright of choice.

You alone can set your eating boundaries.

ple of your sacred self. No one else knows how your body feels, so you alone can set your eating boundaries.

Your emotions are felt by no one as you feel them, and you may well feel them in your solar plexus as hunger. Since they're personal emotions in your private body, only you can separate them and address each feeling individually and appropriately.

A boundary that you choose is achievement—a good and joyous activity—control of your destiny and creativity. But in submitting eating to the achievement model, you try to control it and lose touch with your sensitivity to your body's hunger signals. Thus, you are externalizing an internal signal, hunger.

In submitting eating to the achievement model, you try to control it.

Fear is a natural emotion and serves a purpose. However, when you lose or fail to create internal boundaries, you can develop an unhealthy fear that you lack strength over various aspects of your life, including food. So you seek diets, an external control. By giving away choice, you create a war between your personal need for creating your boundaries and a diet's requirements.

```
┌─ NOTE TO MYSELF ─────────────────────┐
│        I can trust my instincts.      │
└───────────────────────────────────────┘
```

By giving away choice to a diet, your instinct dictates that the diet will fail. Unfortunately, you will probably punish yourself for a very natural conclusion to a boundary skirmish. Specific boundaries are identified and formed (circles) as you take possession of and responsibility for each act of eating. Diets become an irritation because they are unnecessary and have nothing to do with your process. In fact, they work against your process—your personal, private, sacred boundaries.

Diets become an irritation because they are unnecessary and have nothing to do with your process.

If relationships have so overridden your early efforts to form boundaries that the process has been delayed, it's not too late to get started on them. In fact, your eating boundaries are probably just one of the boundary-formation areas that will benefit from your attention.

Experiences such as physical or sexual abuse can be the kind of invasion responsible for eating problems and lack of personal bound-

Overcontrolling parents, as well as experiences in the world that parents have nothing to do with, can contribute to boundary confusion.

aries. But overcontrolling parents, as well as experiences in the world that parents have nothing to do with, can contribute to boundary confusion. Nevertheless, you can regain your boundaries and become a whole, integrated, and self-accepting person by taking back your choices and building healthy boundaries.

Exterior images that come from the culture as ideals to imitate may have discouraged you from accepting your body as a valid size and shape. The healthy boundaries that you are beginning to form will encourage you to choose your personal image and to develop a strong inner system of values. Processing information such as nutrition and physical fitness is something that you will do naturally and comfortably according to your personal, private, and healthy boundaries and values. Making choices will become comfortable for you.

┌─**NOTE TO MYSELF**────────────────────┐

By setting my boundaries, I gain strength.

└──────────────────────────────────────┘

Making choices helps create boundaries, and boundaries further help you to make choices to trust your ability and right to do so. But dependency on exterior controls encourages further dependency. Thus, as you indulge your instinct for health, you will grow stronger.

The instinct you were born with to eat only as much as you need to maintain your health is still in you, alive and well, waiting to be uncovered again. You lost touch with that instinct through boundary invasion of one kind or another. Your restored awareness of the presence and purpose of the feeling of hunger will help you create boundaries that make dependency on external controls impossible.

CHAPTER SUMMARY

The opening Ellis Park story points to the need for boundaries. Establishing boundaries is an old practice in Oriental culture and is important in close-quarter relationships. Families may practice boundary invasion, but adults can build healthy boundaries. Inner Eating aids boundary building and repair relative to voices and scripts and guidance in childhood. The process helps you identify choices and feelings and shows why diets aren't workable. As you learn to do these things, you validate yourself. Healthy boundaries affirm healthy choices.

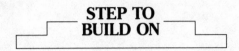

STEP TO
BUILD ON

1. Review the areas where Inner Eating aids boundary building to see which area(s) you want to work on first. Journaling may be beneficial in this process.

Fear/Control

12

Fear of Your Goal

Why, you may ask, would anyone fear a personal goal, especially when it involves something like body size? Have you ever dreamed and fantasized about when you will be able to wear your goal size? Do any of these statements sound familiar?

- Everything will be easier.
- People will respect me more.
- People will like me better.
- I'll be happier.
- I'll be able to wear elegant clothes.
- I'll be sexually acceptable/attractive.
- I can be athletic.
- I won't be embarrassed by my body.
- I can eat in public.
- I won't be so tired.

You may have even felt that those things are more than possibilities; they are promises you make to yourself. Meanwhile, you put them on hold until you reach your "ideal" weight. You haven't yet realized that by respecting and honoring your body now, as you learn its signals and its limits, you can begin to live your dreams now.

By respecting and honoring your body now, you can begin to live your dreams now.

┌─ **NOTE TO MYSELF** ──────────────────┐
│ *I'm going to live my dreams.* │
└──┘

Inner Eating brings you to live in the present moment, beginning now. You can say right now, "I love being who I am, and I love to be able to choose to do the things I love to do. Now. I don't have to wait anymore."

Let's look at the fantasy list again. Allow yourself to experience each feeling now. To accomplish those fantasies, you can begin now to practice and get so good at them that by the time you've reached your healthy state, you'll be an expert at them. That way your mind can keep pace with your body instead of putting your dreams on hold. That can help you release the fear of accepting yourself today because you're afraid you'll give up striving if you do.

Everything will be easier. If life is difficult now, take charge of your time and your day and know that you can make changes today. The more you are in charge of your choices, the easier your life is.

People will respect me more. As you treat your body with greater respect, you'll respect yourself more. You don't have to wait. No one will respect you more than you respect yourself, and you are a most respectable person.

Begin now to practice and get so good at those fantasies that by the time you've reached your healthy state, you'll be an expert at them.

The more you are in charge of your choices, the easier your life is.

┌─ **NOTE TO MYSELF** ──────────────────┐
│ *As I respect myself, so will the world respect me.* │
└──┘

People will like me better. As is the case with respect, liking yourself sets the standard, and who has a better right to respect you than you? After all, you must spend your whole life with you.

┌─ **NOTE TO MYSELF** ──────────────────┐
│ *I need approval from myself and others. So I will* │
│ *approve of myself right now, then others' approval* │
│ *will follow.* │
└──┘

I'll be happier. If you're unhappy about something today, why live with it another day? If you make the decision to be happy today, you'll spend more of your life being happy, and the longer you practice it, the better you'll be at it.

If you make the decision to be happy today, you'll spend more of your life being happy.

┌─**NOTE TO MYSELF**──────────────────────┐
I give myself permission to join the dance of life.
└──────────────────────────────────────┘

I'll be able to wear elegant clothes. Elegance doesn't just happen. It takes a mind-set, practice, and bearing, and the longer you use those skills, the better you'll be at it. So, begin now.

I'll be sexually acceptable/attractive. Sexuality begins in the mind. If someone has treated you unacceptably, forget him or her and look to yourself for acceptance. Don't get hooked by media images of sexuality. Choose your own images.

Don't get hooked by media images of sexuality.

┌─**NOTE TO MYSELF**──────────────────────┐
I am willing to accept love from myself and others.
└──────────────────────────────────────┘

I can be athletic. Once you've had a good physical and are aware of your limitations, begin doing whatever you can do in private or where you feel comfortable. If you begin now, you can accept and claim your muscles and your body, tone your body, and raise your metabolism. Feel free to enjoy movement without fear of judgment. Remember, don't judge yourself. Respect yourself, today and tomorrow.

Feel free to enjoy movement without fear of judgment.

I won't be embarrassed by my body. You don't have to like your body now, but respecting it will help you move toward your goal and will remove a barrier for you. I understand your feeling of embarrassment. I felt it, too. But do everything you can to affirm yourself. You are a person on the move.

I can eat in public. Part of respecting yourself is owning your eating occasions, identifying your beginnings and endings, and making choices. As you become increasingly comfortable with that process, you'll forget to think about what others think because you'll be making your decisions based on your choices.

Don't overdo and hurt yourself. You're not in a race.

I won't be so tired. If you're tired now, take responsibility for it; respect your body's feelings and rest. Exercise to increase your mobility, metabolism, and muscle tone—as you can, listening to your body. Don't overdo and hurt yourself. You're not in a race. You'll find that your energy and enthusiasm—an important factor—are increasing.

By naming your fears today, you disarm them. By facing them and acting on them today, you remove feelings that have been a barrier to living your life now. (See 12-A.)

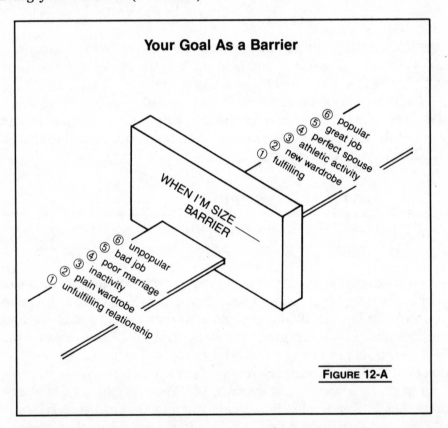

Your Goal As a Barrier

WHEN I'M SIZE ___ BARRIER

① fulfilling
② new wardrobe
③ athletic activity
④ perfect spouse
⑤ great job
⑥ popular

① unfulfilling relationship
② plain wardrobe
③ inactivity
④ poor marriage
⑤ bad job
⑥ unpopular

FIGURE 12-A

Perhaps you have placed a condition on your life. For example, when I reach size 00, I will

- go after that high-paying job.
- get my graduate degree.
- find a spouse.
- go on a dream vacation.

By setting a condition on your dream, you have placed it at a safe distance. Dreams can be scary. Although they promise rewards, they may also mean leaving comfortable and familiar safety. If your body size is a condition, it may also be a safety valve. That is, your dream can't demand anything from you until you meet your condition. Do you see that you may unconsciously hang on to your extra weight because you fear your dream as much as you desire it?

If your body size is a condition, it may also be a safety valve.

Betty Marshall dealt with the issue of her size as both a goal and a barrier. When she reached her goal, she said in surprise, "It's no different from when you're heavier. Thin isn't being perfect, is it?"

You may unconsciously hang on to your extra weight.

"That's true," I agreed. "If you have put conditions on reaching a certain weight, reaching that weight means facing the important issues in your life all at once. If you learn to listen to your body on the way, you can own your body as something uniquely yours all the way along."

The key is involvement in all aspects of being you along the way, the steps you take to gain them, your choices and what you allow to influence those choices, your image, your happiness. Everything that is you is up to you.

Everything that is you is up to you.

If you set conditions for a certain weight, you may also be playing the mind-body game of blaming your body for its refusal to lose weight and dumping on it the responsibility for all your troubles, rejections, and pain.

I see three reasons—and there are probably more—why some people may have body size barriers. First, fat symbolizes something else. It can be a wall that keeps others out, a wall that protects against unacceptable feelings.

Second, fat can maintain focus on the weight instead of the real issue, the primary problem. (For a discussion of this, see chapter 9.)

Third, fat acts as a built-in saboteur. The words *saboteur* and *sabotage* come from a wooden shoe, the sabot, worn by workers in early French factories. When they wanted to protest, one of their sabots "fell" into the machinery. Thus, you sabotage yourself with accidents and excuses that prevent weight loss, for fear of the consequences once you attain a certain size. Reasons vary, and they're done unconsciously, but they are a barrier.

You sabotage yourself with accidents and excuses that prevent weight loss.

Margaret, for example, stayed thirty pounds overweight for years, although she tried lots of diets. One day she admitted that when she was thin, men flirted with her or made passes at her. She feared she might have been leading them on, so she decided not to be so enticing and put on weight.

Her grandfather had railed against "loose and immoral women, and females dressing and acting provocatively just to lead men to destruction." Later Margaret learned that he was a womanizer, and his noise was nothing but a defensive smoke screen. She remembered overhearing him say to her grandmother, "I wouldn't ever chase after women if they didn't behave the way they do." Margaret adored her grandfather, and she never questioned his twisted reasoning. She grew up determined not to lead men astray. Staying overweight kept her from "leading men down the wrong road."

Linda Kemp feared being thin. She discovered that she hadn't really learned much about nutrition, choice, or taste, despite having been on twenty different diets. When the diets got her to her goal weight, she was afraid that she couldn't stay there because she didn't know *how* she got there. The diets gave her no understanding. She knew how to be overweight, but she didn't know how to be thin.

Dan has been corpulent all of his life. He has tried and failed at a dozen diets. Only when he began to look beyond his bulky image did he start to understand himself.

Dan came from a family with a domineering parent who wouldn't allow the three children to raise their voices. "We don't get angry. We forgive."

Dan felt anger often, but he stuffed it down with food. Eating made him feel better when his anger became overwhelming.

He married a woman who did not believe in anger. "I refuse to allow other people to upset me," she said. Dan listened, and ate, and kept getting heavier. At age forty-one he recognized the cause of his weight. "It's easier to stay fat than to confront my wife and my mother." He could just as well add, "It's also easier to stay fat than to own the fact that I'm angry. If I admit I'm angry, I have to take responsibility for my anger."

Jim Burton is an active member of ACOA (Adult Children of Alcoholics). As he approached middle age, Jim connected his extra weight with his alcoholic family background. He wanted "friendship and real intimacy with other people," but he was afraid. As a child in a dysfunctional family, he couldn't depend on or trust his parents. Until just recently Jim has had difficulty trusting anyone else. "My fat body," he said, "was my protective wall against anyone getting too close."

Body image and ownership is also an intensely defended issue for people who have experienced childhood sexual abuse. They may go two ways. They may maintain a barrier of weight as a defense, even going so far as to make themselves as unattractive as possible, but without ever realizing why they do so. Or they may refuse to eat, staying dangerously thin, avoiding maturation and development of secondary sex characteristics in an effort to avoid adult sexuality. In short, they're afraid to grow up because adulthood means sexuality to them, and sexuality means invasion, pain, fear, and helplessness. In such cases, Inner Eating, learning to identify and honor the body's needs, is often a path to partial recovery, with therapy completing the process.

Like Margaret, like Linda, like Dan, like Jim, you may be unconsciously setting up barriers. As I pointed out in chapter 9, body size isn't the real issue; defense is. If you continue to concentrate on weight and losing pounds, you are throwing your own sabot into the machinery. You're then continuing to look at the weight when something deeper may be more important. Only you can know if and why you have a barrier. But there needn't be a barrier at all if you concentrate on respecting your body at each eating occasion and live today. If there is to be a goal, respecting your body is the goal—and how can one be fearful of that?

If you're afraid of reaching your goal weight, your reasons are probably unconscious.

CHAPTER SUMMARY

You may be afraid of losing weight because you have set conditions on a certain weight. By taking charge of your choices and behavior now, you can build strength while you work toward your dreams. By living in the present, life becomes more fully realized, and the future no longer threatens. There are at least three reasons people create barriers: protection, focus, and sabotage. Margaret stayed overweight to lessen her sexual attractiveness; Linda knew only how to be "fat"; Dan ate to stuff his anger rather than face it; Jim used fat for protection against betrayal. Some people use excess weight as protection against sexual abuse. If there is to be a goal, then the goal would be to respect your body at each eating occasion.

STEPS TO
BUILD ON

1. Identify and write in your journal about any issue or issues that sabotage your efforts to listen to your body's signals.

2. Consider getting Susan Jeffers' *Feel the Fear and Do It Anyway*, which discusses the particular problem(s) that block you, to help you be fully informed and equipped.

13

Fear of Fat

Sixteen-year-old Chiara feared becoming fat, which is why she sought my help. She was a gymnast, and her gymnastic activities were ending for the season, so she would have a few weeks off. She ate very little, and I thought it was amazing that she could perform so well with the small amount of energy she supplied her body.

"If I eat more, I get sick," Chiara said. The very thought of food raised the specter of fat for her so strongly that she had rejected her body. She believed that eating even normal amounts would make her fat. Whenever any significant amount of food went into her body, she became uncomfortable emotionally.

The very thought of food raised the specter of fat for her.

A high achiever, and a good athlete who was not the least bit overweight, Chiara looked like an attractive, well-toned young woman. Yet her appearance wasn't as important as how she felt about her body. When we started talking about eating, I asked, "What does food mean to you?"

Her appearance wasn't as important as how she felt about her body.

"Getting fat."

Then I asked, "What do you think when you see somebody eat pizza?"

"You're crazy to eat pizza. You're going to get fat."

Although I asked several other questions, she had already made her problem clear. For Chiara, food represented fat. Eating only tiny amounts of certain foods meant staying thin. She feared she'd give in,

She found no enjoyment in eating.

binge, and gain weight. Consequently, she feared food, and she found no enjoyment in eating or in caring for her body.

As I listened, I thought, *How can you care for something you hate or you feel such disgust for?*

I asked her, "What do you feel like when you're wearing your leotards and you're standing there, getting ready to go on for the floor routine? What feelings do you have just before you start your routine?"

"I feel fat," she said.

"Okay," I said, "and once you get into your routine, what do you feel like?"

"I'm performing then. I'm not thinking about my body," she said.

Her body was a means to achievement.

Her attitude was fairly obvious. Since she put everything into her performance, her body was a means to achievement. When Chiara came off the floor, she was back to herself, and she hated her body.

When I've mentioned this self-hatred, listeners are usually surprised. Someone will usually ask, "Why wouldn't gymnasts like their bodies? Aren't they in tune with their bodies? Wouldn't they be the first people in the world to take care of their bodies?"

That may sound logical, yet it doesn't work that way with people like Chiara. Because she demanded perfection of herself, she lived with the fear of getting fat. She was afraid that one occasion of overeating would cause her to hate her body. She worked at maintaining the perfect image.

She was unaware of hunger or any other feelings that would validate her core self.

As a result, Chiara felt like a hollow person. Her shell (perfect self) was the obedient child, the performer, the exceller, the lovely girl. Her core self was empty. She focused so intently on her shell (perfect self) that she was unaware of her core self. And since hunger is felt in the core self, she was unaware of hunger or any other feelings that would validate her core self. Chiara needed a blending, an integration of her selves into a validated wholeness.

I knew I had to help Chiara understand her separation. Then together we could break through the mind-set that kept her from normal eating. The simplest way to start was to ask her about her body and find out what she considered so bad about it to get to her real feelings. If we could break through, I knew she could start caring for her body and work on the issue of food.

"You can choose to take charge of your life. Or you can choose to let fear hold you."

"You have choices," I said. "You always have choices. You can choose to get rid of fear. You can choose to take charge of your life. Or you can choose to let fear hold you. Are you willing to take risks so you can move beyond fear?"

"Yes, I really am!"

"What about your eating would you like to change?"

"My erratic eating pattern," Chiara said.

"Why?"

"Because when I do give in, I eat too much. And I'm afraid."

"Afraid of what?" I asked.

"Of getting fat."

"Let's try an exercise," I said to Chiara. "Just relax. Close your eyes. Think of yourself now. Picture what you look like when I tell you that you're now at the weight you like. It's the perfect weight for you."

When she had the image in mind, I said, "This is the weight you will always be. No matter how much you eat, you will never get fat. You won't get thinner, either. You'll always remain at this perfect weight for you."

This has proved to be a most useful method to help others move beyond fear. I wanted to show Chiara what her eating pattern would be without fear filling her mind.

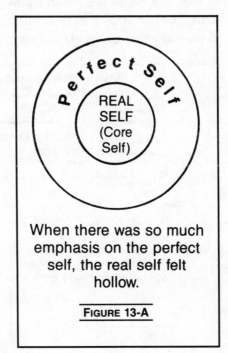

When there was so much emphasis on the perfect self, the real self felt hollow.

FIGURE 13-A

"No matter how much you eat, you will never get fat."

"Now, Chiara, you are at the weight you always wanted to be. Your body is perfect. It will always stay that way, regardless of the amount of food or the kind of food. Now tell me, how you would eat?"

"Now tell me, how you would eat?"

"I would eat more regularly."

"Would you eat a ton of food?"

"No, of course not."

"Then what is the fear doing for you?"

Suddenly her face glowed with insight. "Fear is causing me to eat erratically. This fear makes me eat less, and it's causing me to hate my body. Then I get mad and eat too much."

"If you could get rid of the fear, how would your life change? If you eliminated the fear and the hatred of the body, and learned regular eating habits that you felt good with, how would that change your life?"

"I could really live my life," Chiara said. "I could be less stressful."

"So the goal is to get rid of this fear of fat. Is that it?"

"Yes," she said. "That's what I want."

The fear of fat was causing her erratic eating behavior and her stress.

Although this is just a summary, we went through several exercises so that she could see clearly how strong her fear of being fat and her hatred of her body had become. She had to see for herself that the fear of fat was causing her erratic eating behavior and her stress. (See 13-B.)

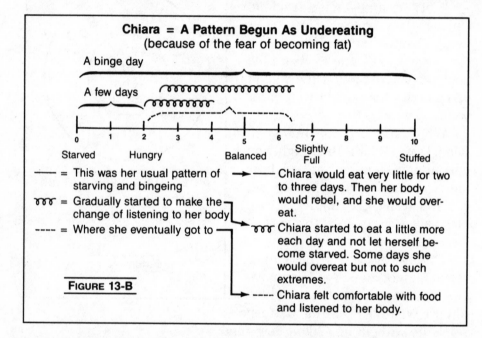

"Let's do another exercise," I said. "What do you hate about your body? Tell me six things that you dislike intensely about your body. Remember, Chiara, food really isn't the issue in your situation. So what do you hate?"

"I hate my body. All of it."

"Okay. Now, let's be specific. Name one thing about your body you don't like."

"All right. I hate my hair."

"Now let's have a second thing you hate about your body."

As Chiara talked about her body, I could see only a beautiful and talented girl. Finally she said, "I hate my face, my height, my personality. I hate that I'm Filipino."

"Okay, those are the things you hate. What are two things you like?" She couldn't think of anything about her body that she liked, so I asked her to go beyond her body to other things that she might like.

"Achievement." After thinking a little bit she added, "I like my friends."

I said, "Okay, you've told me you hate your body, hair, face, height, and personality. You also hate it that you're Filipino. That's six." Again, anyone who hadn't heard her speak that way would never have dreamed how she felt. At that stage, it wouldn't have helped for me to say, "You've got a beautiful body and beautiful hair."

I turned to what she liked. There was nothing about herself, so we moved beyond to her achievement. "You like to achieve, but you've actually taken yourself out of your life. You've given yourself to achievement and to friends. You don't even have a place for you in your life. The more of yourself you take out of what you have, the bigger the hole, the deeper the emptiness. That's a horrible feeling."

"You've given yourself to achievement and to friends. You don't even have a place for you in your life."

Tears filled her eyes, and she nodded; she truly understood her emptiness.

"Do you feel the emptiness?"

"Yes."

"This is what we're going to work on," I said, "because you've taken you out of yourself. So let's look at this information more closely. Let's see what's so bad about it. I want you to do another exercise with me. This time you have to make choices. Choose between your body and your hair. You can't say they're equal."

"This time you have to make choices."

We went through all of the things she didn't like. I was taking her through a grid of choices, as I've done with others. (See chapter 4.)

GRID OF CHOICES

(4)	1. Body	① 2								
(2)	2. Hair	1 ③	2 ③							
(5)	3. Face	① 4	② 4	③ 4						
(2)	4. Height	① 5	② 5	③ 5	④ 5					
(0)	5. Personality	① 6	2 6	③ 6	④ 6	5 ⑥				
(1)	6. Filipino									

On the first line are the numbers 1 and 2. I asked her to compare her body and her hair. "Which do you hate more?"

When she said her body, I circled number 1. Then she compared her body and her face. I circled the one she disliked more. We continued through the grid until we had compared each item against the others.

When we finished, I went back and counted the number of circles for 1, for 2, and so on.

(If you do this, in case two numbers have the same number of circles, go back to the grid and see which one you circled when you compared those two.)

When we had finished, Chiara had the fewest circles around 5. Personality.

"You said that your personality really isn't so bad. Right?"

She nodded.

"Then why don't you take your personality back? You said it's not so bad."

Being Filipino was next. "Take that back. Own that. You yourself said it's not so bad being Filipino."

She had made all the choices. I was showing her that she could own those qualities.

She had made all the choices. I was showing her that she could own those qualities.

The one with the most circles was her face. I said, "Okay, what is it about your face that you don't like?"

She said, "My eyes, my nose, the texture, the shape, my mouth, and the color." We went through a grid again, listing each quality.

Again, when we finished, we counted circles. A couple of them didn't even get circled. "So you can take those back, can't you? They aren't so bad. You can own those." She had chosen her nose as her worst feature.

"Models emphasize what's good."

"Chiara, we've come down to your nose. Now I have another question. Do models emphasize what's bad?"

"No, they emphasize what's good."

"You're right," I said. "Do you think there's any perfect model? Anyone who doesn't have some area they compensate for?"

"No," she said, "probably not."

I told Chiara about a friend, Carroll Britton, who does makeup. I said, "I'd like to make an appointment, and we'll go over there. She'll show you what she does with makeup and shading"

I set it up, and my friend did a wonderful job of shading Chiara's face. Chiara wanted a narrower nose, and my friend made it look that way through contour makeup.

When we met again, Chiara started to take back the things that she had said she hated.

"What's your feeling when you look at people who can see only their bad qualities, while you can look at them and see so many good ones?"

"I feel that it's such a waste of time for those people."

As I continued to work with Chiara, she was able to see what she was doing to herself. She realized she needed to emphasize the good and diminish the bad.

You may wonder why I spent so much time going through the exercises. Chiara had such a strong hatred of her body that she was blocked. Once I could help her deal with the real issue of her fear of fat, we could begin to work on her eating. Only then could we start with the circles of eating.

Chiara had such a strong hatred of her body that she was blocked.

————————————— ☐ —————————————

The real work started when she thought about caring for her body, and not rejecting it before she ate.

I've taken this chapter to tell you one person's story. Yet Chiara isn't so different from others. She had an athletic and trim body, but what good did it do her? Because of self-hatred of her body, she could have weighed three times as much and wouldn't have felt any different.

┌─**NOTE TO MYSELF**─────────────────────┐

Eating isn't a matter of fat or thin. Eating is to take care of my body.

└──────────────────────────────────────┘

When I first help clients confront their fear, it may be the biggest block they face. It may be fear of food or fear of something else that they use food to cover. That's where the grid exercise takes the teeth out of the fear. Maybe fear of fat is your problem, and you label foods fattening or nonfattening, good or bad.

Can you see what happens when you get caught up in fear? If you slip up and eat a "bad" food, you transfer that feeling to yourself and begin to think of yourself as a bad person.

If so much depends on being thin, it makes sense why so many people are afraid of doing anything that will make them fat.

The image of what you want your body to be is the illusion that distorts your sensitivity and sense of ownership of your body. This difference may appear slight, but it creates many problems. The illusion comes from the idea that being thinner makes everything fine. If so much depends on being thin, it makes sense why so many people are afraid of doing anything that will make them fat.

Along with this, fear works in another way. Soon you decide that if you don't cut out certain foods or cut down the amounts, you're bound to get very fat. Chiara thought that not eating to get thin would also keep her thin. Actually, that kind of thinking created her erratic eating pattern.

The body will take voluntary deprivation only so long.

With Chiara, as well as with others, the severe food restriction caused her to binge later. As I've pointed out elsewhere, the body will take voluntary deprivation only so long. Then it rebels.

"The more you think about fat and thin instead of listening to your body," I told Chiara, "the farther you move away from your body. The more you move away from your body, the less able you are to hear the messages you need."

Once the nibbling began, she didn't stop until she had binged.

Here's Chiara's typical eating pattern. She tried not to eat breakfast and lunch—she wasn't listening to her body. For about three days she could hold out, refusing to hear her body signals. By the fourth day, she would start to nibble. Once the nibbling began, she didn't stop until she had binged.

After Chiara explained her erratic eating, I tried to sum up for her what was happening. "For three days," I said, "you let your head take over. You ate practically nothing. Finally the body rebelled and took over, and you ate too much. What were you thinking when you were bingeing?"

"That I lacked willpower," she said.

Lack of willpower makes it an issue of self-blame.

That's the usual response I get to that question. Lack of willpower makes it an issue of self-blame.

"Now that you're over this binge," I said, "what would you normally do about eating?"

"I'd try harder."

Chiara and many others get caught in this cycle of not listening to their bodies, so they fight against themselves. When they binge, they blame themselves for being weak and unable to stop their eating. Once they finish that cycle of overeating, they make new resolutions to be stricter—exert more willpower. So the cycle begins again and won't end until they just give up in self-disgust.

Some people with whom I've worked tell me they put off eating breakfast and lunch—what I call operating in their heads. That is, they decide not to eat without considering the needs and demands of their bodies. Then sometime in the afternoon the body rebels and the binge-ing starts. Some have said, "I was under so much stress, I just gave in and ate."

Some people decide not to eat without consider-ing the needs and de-mands of their bodies.

Stress is a reality and may be a serious problem. Yet too many people say, "I feel stressed. Consequently, I eat." Stress, or any emotion or problem, is a separate issue from eating, and I urge these people to recognize that.

Individuals who fear fat don't think of hunger as a message from their bodies. How can they? They're fighting their bodies.

Somewhat along this same line, Colette Dowling refers to Dr. Hilda Bruch's book, *Eating Disorders:*

Dr. Hilda Bruch tells us the problem begins in early childhood. It's important, as we grow up, for us to learn to "code," or make use of messages coming from our bodies. That is the only way we can learn to identify bodily needs and satisfy them. Thus, Bruch emphasizes, if a girl is going to be able to take care of herself, she needs to know what her body is feeling. Only when a mother offers food in response to signals indicating nutritional need, says Bruch, will the infant grad-ually develop the engram of "hunger" as a sensation distinct from other tensions and needs.[1]

NOTE TO MYSELF

Fear of fat and fat-thin thinking separate me from my body.

Internal dialogue that addresses the fat-thin image but doesn't consider eating for the reason of hunger has negative results. (See 13-C.) When you listen to your body, you own and enjoy each circle of eating. Then the statements are positive, with no self-judgments or self-recriminations. Consequently, your day can flow easier with consistent spurts of energy.

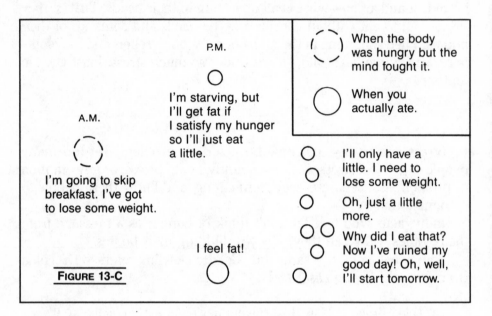

FIGURE 13-C

If you are caught in the trap of hearing chatter or old tapes inside your head, making you afraid of getting fat, you can change them. When you hear the script inside your head saying the words in the left column, you can stop the recording. Here are a few substitute statements.

THESE STATEMENTS MAY CAUSE ERRATIC EATING PATTERNS:	THESE STATEMENTS WILL HELP YOU CHANGE THE RECORDING:
"Oh, I feel fat. I'd better cut down tomorrow."	"Wait. How does my body feel now?"
"I'd better not eat that. It might make me fat."	"Is this the food I like? Is it nutritious?"
"Oh, to be like that thin model, I'd have to starve."	"This is my body. I don't have to look like anyone else."

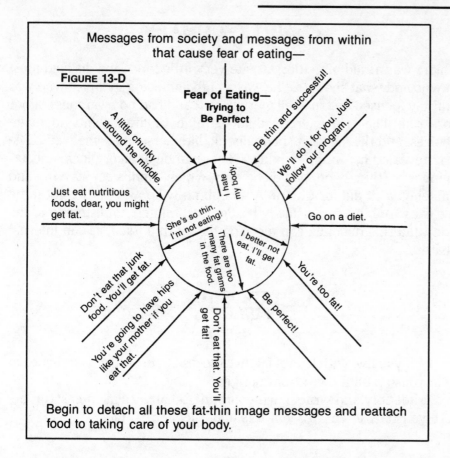

Messages from society and messages from within that cause fear of eating—

FIGURE 13-D

**Fear of Eating—
Trying to
Be Perfect**

Be thin and successful!

We'll do it for you. Just follow our program.

A little chunky around the middle.

I hate my body.

Just eat nutritious foods, dear, you might get fat.

She's so thin. I'm not eating!

Go on a diet.

There are too many fat grams in the food.

I better not eat. I'll get fat.

Don't eat that junk food. You'll get fat.

You're going to have hips like your mother if you eat that.

Don't eat that. You'll get fat!

Be perfect!

You're too fat!

Begin to detach all these fat-thin image messages and reattach food to taking care of your body.

As I've already pointed out, the fear of fat and the desire to be thin cause erratic eating patterns. You may feel that if you loosen the tight restrictions, you'll get fat. I hope you'll be able to realize that such an attitude may be keeping you fat or in an unhealthy relationship with food.

Remember, you can establish your own eating habits by changing your mental attitude and the script that is going on in your head. When you decide to change any pattern of behavior, be aware that experts say it takes about four weeks of vigilance before you can consider that you've made a permanent change. Be patient with yourself.

┌─**NOTE TO MYSELF**─────────────
│ *Fear of fat blocks my hunger signals.*
└──────────────────────────────

CHAPTER SUMMARY

Chiara was afraid of getting fat, ate very little food, and disliked most of who and what she was. She was a high-achieving gymnast who was entirely focused on her shell (perfect self) and had no awareness of her core self. The grid exercise demonstrated Chiara's ability to make choices, and the fact that she really did like herself in some ways. The grid revealed her inner emptiness. Fear can be a major block, encouraging a fat/thin, good/bad dichotomy, which can trigger starving and bingeing, as it did for Chiara. Although no willpower is thought to be the cause of bingeing, actually it's deprivation and not listening to the body. Internal dialogue can focus on the fat-thin issue, as can internal chatter.

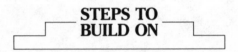

STEPS TO BUILD ON

1. If you live with fear of fat, use the grid to prioritize your issues to help you separate them from hunger.

2. Identify and write down your inner chatter/dialogue/script before you start to eat to see if it is about fear or hunger.

NOTE

1. Colette Dowling, *Perfect Women* (New York: Pocket Books, 1988), p. 111.

14

The Issue of Control

Self-control is often regarded as the missing element in overeating problems. On the other hand, anorexics and bulimics have an enormous problem with overcontrol. In my opinion, control creates the problems, along with the presence of unrelated issues that affect the eating pattern. A healthy eating pattern is a form of self-respect, not self-control. When I think of Jon's eating pattern, I realize that he doesn't use control; he just respects his body by listening to his hunger signals. He doesn't try to control his amounts, nor even think about control. He has created a healthy eating pattern by respecting his body.

Developing a personal healthy eating pattern involves identifying unrelated issues, understanding and respecting the body, and letting go of control. Think about a time when you aren't hungry, when there are no signals from your body telling you to eat. Remember and respect that feeling and be responsible to yourself to find an activity appropriate to the moment other than eating, even if it's just relaxing.

A healthy eating pattern is a form of self-respect, not self-control.

———————————— □ ————————————

Bonnie, whom I mentioned earlier, had been using the Inner Eating process for about two years. When her mother became suddenly and debilitatingly ill, Bonnie was overwhelmed. Her helplessness and pain overrode the stability she had achieved, and she returned to eating as an action—doing something, anything—in an uncontrollable situation.

When her mother began to recover—without benefit from Bonnie's eating, I might add—Bonnie was unhappy about the extra weight she had gained. We talked, and she became aware of the dynamics of her eating behavior. She returned to listening to her body, a true form of self-respect, and stabilized her weight again.

Eating doesn't control anything but your hunger.

The point, again, is obvious. Eating for any reason other than hunger does nothing for anything outside the body. Eating doesn't control anything but your hunger. The feeling of control for eaters comes from the fact that they're at least taking some action, no matter how inappropriate to the problem at hand.

Someone who doesn't know about the Inner Eating process may well turn to dieting as a form of control. But he or she will create another problem by substituting one form of powerlessness for another.

Peter Vash of *Shape* commented on the magazine's survey on why people diet. His data

> suggest that respondents are clinging to a host of dietary contradictions that shortchange them emotionally as well as nutritionally. Instead of developing life skills that would give them true power over their lives, they resort to dieting as a symbolic form of self-control.[1]

You may be convinced that if you let go, everything will fall apart.

You may like to be in control of every situation—many of us do. You may try to control another person because you sincerely believe it's for his or her own good. You feel the need, and the responsibility, to hold things together in your home. You may be convinced that if you let go, everything will fall apart.

However, Dr. Cloud shows how that control affects others.

> When people are denied ownership of their behavior and the consequences for it, they feel enormously powerless. A false dependency is created that leaves them with no sense of security in their ability to cause an effect.[2]

There are people who are enormously competent and self-assured but who feel inadequate to control their eating, and so they turn to diet programs. These people then depend on someone else to weigh them and to make them responsible for their eating.

The false dependency mentioned by Dr. Cloud reminds me of the time Elaine Leff and I were talking about dieting and weight control at a tennis party. Previously she had been on the Weight Watchers program. She felt it was the best program for her, and she had decided to rejoin the program. "Now I can eat right and eat healthy foods," she said.

When she mentioned eating right, I asked her several questions. "Do you know about the four food groups?"

"Oh, yes," she answered. "And I've learned what my body needs."

As we talked more about nutrition, Elaine said, "I know all of that backward and forward." And she did.

"Elaine," I asked, "if you know all of that, why do you need an external control? Why do you need someone to weigh you?"

She looked surprised. "I don't know. I know when food feels good in my body, and I know what amounts my body needs. So why do I need someone else to put me on the scales?"

I didn't answer, because I sensed that Elaine was in the process of letting go of her need for an external control and forming internal boundaries.

Quite aptly, Dr. Cloud writes, "Our sense of being able to own our behavior is critical for having a sense of power over our lives and a sense of self-control."[3] External control throws instinct off balance. The scales are a form of external control.

Elaine was in the process of letting go of external boundaries and forming internal boundaries.

The Scales

The bathroom scale has become a permanent piece of furniture in most homes, and most people weigh themselves automatically. Some people become so compulsive that they weigh five or six times a day, every day. Or they weigh every time they finish eating. Sadly, a heavy reliance on scales really works against you. Here's why.

Scales rob you of an honest relationship with your body. At a time when you're trying to get in touch with your body, weighing yourself encourages you to rely on the scale rather than your body's signals.

Scales make judgments about you. You feel judged as a person and as a body according to where the dial marker points. This balancing machine decides whether you're a good person or a bad one.

Scales dictate and control. When you weigh, the results hint that if you're good today, maybe you can cheat—a little bit anyway. Or if you overate yesterday, you must cut back drastically today.

Scales rob you of your ability to stay in tune with your body. You can't concentrate on the pleasure of eating; you're too busy calculating amounts.

Scales set the emotional tone for the day. If your weight is up, you're cranky and depressed. If it's down, you relax and enjoy life a little.

Scales keep you in fear. Even if you have five good days in a row (i.e., your weight is down), always lurking in your mind is the fear of letting up, of gaining weight, of failing, of wondering if you ate too much pizza, or if you should have stopped with a single slice of bread.

Scales teach you to say negative things to yourself, such as:

"I weighed three pounds too much today, so I can't eat this. Maybe by Friday, if I'm good . . ."

"I can't make choices. I have to be strict."

"I weigh too much, and I'm ugly."

"I can't deal with my emotions because my weight is up. When I'm fourteen pounds lighter, I'll be able to concentrate on other things."

"The scale is up today. Another bad day for me."

Or you play games with the scales:

- You step sideways on the scales.
- You take off everything that can possibly count as weight, including rings.
- You make sure you go to the bathroom first.
- You weigh the first thing in the morning, before you put an ounce of anything in your system.
- You put scales on a rug, and move around a little to manipulate a lower reading.

In short, the scales control you because you've given the scales control.

Bill weighed in at 212 and said, "Until I am 170, I can't be happy."

Margaret read the figure of 122 and sighed, "Until I'm 115, I can't go to any social event."

Or you say, "When I weigh X pounds, I'll be able to wear my new suit."

"When I weigh X pounds, I'll reward myself with a coconut cake."

I don't weigh my clients because the number they see inhibits their inner growth. When weight is the focus, they get stuck there and fail to identify and resolve the issues that affected the eating that caused the extra weight. The issues need to be the focus; the weight loss is a by-product. Success is hearing the following statements:

"It's so nice not to care about the scale."

"I'm not on a weight yo-yo anymore."

"Eating is no longer my major activity."

"I don't need to eat as much as I thought I did."

"I don't have to be afraid of hunger. I know I can listen to my body."

"My clothes fit so well, and all I had to do was respect my body."

Consuming food as a form of control over circumstances or over others doesn't work, as we have seen. On the other hand, not consuming food as a tool of self-control is a method others use to the point that the rigidity of the program controls them. In short, they lose control over their control.

The pattern of bulimics is to go from extremes of control to out of control.

The pattern of bulimics is to go from extremes of control to out of control. They use tight control such as extreme dieting because they fear getting fat. Control causes a sense of deprivation which may combine true food deprivation with feelings of emptiness caused by other nonfood issues. The resulting binge goes out of control because it feeds a physical and emotional need. Once the physical and emotional emptiness is filled, the control requirement reasserts itself. Bulimics purge, and control is reestablished. Purging uses one or a variety of forms of catharsis: vomiting, laxatives, diuretics, enemas, and abusive exercising. Each extreme of the pattern is brief. Bulimics range between the extremes of eating and not eating, but anorexics refuse to eat. In both cases the issue is self-control to the point of self-destruction.

Anorexics refuse to eat.

Inner Eating has helped bulimics and anorexics regain balance between self-control and eating issues.

┌─ **NOTE TO MYSELF** ─────────────────────┐
│ *Healthy boundaries promote healthy decisions.* │
└──┘

Although not with the same severity, many people who struggle with their weight get caught up in the issue of control by restricting themselves. I think of the time Hillary first talked to me about facing a long table of desserts. She said, "I have this feeling that if I had no restrictions, I'd want everything on the table and totally lose control."

"Hillary," I said, "when you respond to fear of not being able to control your eating, you're not thinking about tasting the food. The way for you to take charge is to choose what you will eat, identify your body signal, and respect that message." And as we saw in chapter 4, she was able to make choices and enjoy eating.

"If you get rid of your self-imposed restric-tions, eventually your body signals will start to tell you when, what, and how much to eat."

At a conference I attended in California in 1989, Jane Hirschmann, who coauthored *Overcoming Overeating* and *Solving Your Child's Eating Problems,* advocated bringing everything you want to eat into the house. "Don't hide it away," she said, "or stop buying it." She was saying that if you get rid of your self-imposed restrictions, eventually your body signals will start to tell you when, what, and how much to eat. Trust your body signals, your instincts, to give you true inner control.

———————————— □ ————————————

Perfectionists and top achievers seem to have more of an issue of control than others.

Who are the people most inclined to fall into the trap of control? Studies show that perfectionists and top achievers seem to have more of an issue of control than others.

The authors of *Love Hunger: Recovery from Food Addiction* wrote,

Control is a major issue, especially to the perfectionist. Most perfectionists are oldest children who grew up in a home where they were overly controlled. In fact, many of the people we treat for obsessive-compulsive disorders are oldest children who have been overly controlled by new parents, anxious to do a good job. A majority of people who excel in science, music, or professional athletics are firstborns. . . .

Control is also a big issue for a child growing up in an unhealthy family. In a dysfunctional family with an alcoholic parent or where there are sexual, physical, or emotional abuses, the child grows up learning to be scared. In defense, they take control of their lives to protect themselves from pain.

"It's not unusual for a binge eater to become a binge spender or a compulsive gambler."

As the child grows older, there are only a few battlegrounds where they can practice their control. Money is one of them. It's not unusual for a binge eater to become a binge spender or a compulsive gambler.

Or, frequently, food becomes the battleground where the perfectionistic person seeks to be the boss over something. In reality, binge eaters aren't in control because the food is in control and is killing them. But they feel as if they're the boss. . . .

Ironically, most compulsive eaters are overdisciplined. They tell themselves, "If I just had more willpower I could beat this food issue. I could make that diet work with a little more willpower." Yet willpower is not the answer. Believing you can solve the problem with just a little more self-control often leads to binge eating each time this faulty approach fails.[4]

Some controllers are *codependent*. That word refers to "destructive and behavioral patterns that develop from prolonged exposure to an oppressive way of life."[5]

In a devotional book called *Keeping My Balance*, Cecil Murphey writes about the way codependency functions:

An oxymoron is a combination of two contradictory words like dull shine. Controlling love is an oxymoron too. The two words don't go together. In the name of love I tried to push, pull, drag, nag, teach, advise, placate, and set straight. When she argued (and she nearly always did), I backed off and sulked. "I was only trying to help because I love you."

I didn't have an addiction, so obviously I knew better than she did what she needed. I also felt that I had to stop her pain. If I didn't do it, nobody would. I knew I was right, and that meant she had to be wrong.

"I love her so much," I consoled myself. "I want her free." I did love her, but I didn't act lovingly. I acted like a benevolent dictator. And I wondered why I always lost.[6]

"I knew I was right, and that meant she had to be wrong."

Controllers tend to be scared people. Manipulating others is their weapon against being hurt. They tend to be overly disciplined. Of those I see, some of them restrain everything else in their lives except their eating. They feel frustrated and powerless. They can't figure out why they have such a problem with food.

Feelings of superiority and inferiority can be an issue for people who have a problem with control. If life is a road, superiority and inferiority are the names of the ditches on either side. They're places to fall

They can't figure out why they have such a problem with food.

into that have nothing to do with getting on with the journey of life. (See 14-A.)

They want to be richest, smartest, thinnest, prettiest, strongest, most creative, sexiest, and so on. They travel along in the ditch of superiority until someone brighter, thinner, or sexier comes along, and then they're dumped into the opposite ditch of inferiority. So they eat to feed the feeling of inferiority.

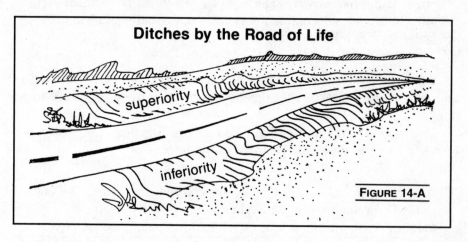

Ditches by the Road of Life

superiority

inferiority

FIGURE 14-A

When food is an issue and it's used to feed the feeling, Inner Eating tools create awareness of actions and healthy alternatives. Using these tools, the former controller can learn to value his or her gifts and the gifts of others as complementary and nonthreatening. Recognition of choices and boundaries affirms personhood and gifts as unique. (See 14-B.)

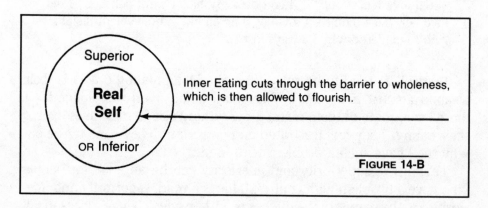

Superior

Real Self

OR Inferior

Inner Eating cuts through the barrier to wholeness, which is then allowed to flourish.

FIGURE 14-B

┌─ NOTE TO MYSELF ─────────────────────────────┐
│   *My gifts complement yours.*   │
└───┘

Our relationships with others—whether in the workplace or the home—may influence us in the issue of control. We may choose to be in charge or look to others to be in charge. These issues may affect our relationship with eating.

We may choose to be in charge or look to others to be in charge.

For persons in power positions, the power has been a positive force, a thing of which they're proud. Yet when they are unable to exert that same power (control) over eating, they are highly frustrated. They try to control their eating without listening to their instincts. Whenever their instincts do win out, they believe they have failed. They can handle everything at work, so why can't they control their eating? They resent the need to submit to external control, such as a diet plan.

Other persons may feel comfortable letting someone else be in charge. If their eating seems out of control, they may, at first, find it easier to let someone else make the decisions. Eventually, however, they start to want to make their own choices—yet feel obligated to follow the plan. Again, when those instincts win out, it feels like a failure.

Trying to control or letting someone else control takes away the freedom to listen to our bodies. Yet we view it as a failure.

If diets have been a failure point for you, consider the probability that you have, at some level, been defying the external control. You've been demonstrating, by your eating in defiance of the diet plan, that no one and nothing is going to tell you what to eat! Consequently, in your own body you have been waging a war of wills, with your body as the battlefield and eating as your weapon.

In your own body you have been waging a war of wills.

If you have fought the control over food, lost control, and punished yourself, and you don't want to remain in that pattern, you are now aware that those two extremes form the external limits of control. In the center of those extremes lies Inner Eating, which empowers you to claim your eating through informed choice.

You no longer have to feel scared, uncertain, and out of control. The self-respect you seek comes to you through the tools of circles, the Hunger Rating Scale, and your boundaries.

The self-control you seek comes to you through the tools of circles, the Hunger Rating Scale, and your boundaries.

---NOTE TO MYSELF---

My self-respect is my ultimate expression of inner strength.

CHAPTER SUMMARY

Choice and self-directed action are the best bases for healthy eating boundaries, whereas diets frustrate control. Eating and dieting for control are actions disconnected from hunger and body signals. Denied ownership of the body creates false dependency; self-respect comes from choosing your own behavior. High achievers are often people with control issues. Compulsive eaters are often overdisciplined people. Codependents are controllers. Superiority and inferiority are ditches on either side of life's road. Food is neutral; control and healthy eating are the issues.

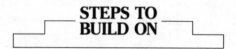

STEPS TO BUILD ON

1. Each time you reach for food today, take a moment to check the Hunger Rating Scale and your stress quotient, and identify your eating trigger.

2. When you eat today, check the impact of others on your eating pattern. Ask yourself, What happens inside me when this other person is around? What does this other person do or say that makes me want to turn to food? Am I the controller? When my controls don't work, do I turn to food?

3. Decide if you want your hunger signals or someone outside yourself to determine your hunger boundaries.

NOTES

1. Peter D. Vash, "Why We Diet," *Shape*, July 1989, p. 84.

2. Henry Cloud, *When Your World Makes No Sense* (Nashville: Oliver-Nelson Books, 1990), p. 112.

3. Cloud, *When Your World Makes No Sense*, p. 147.

4. Frank Minirth, Paul Meier, Robert Hemfelt, and Sharon Sneed, *Love Hunger: Recovery from Food Addiction* (Nashville: Oliver-Nelson Books, 1990), pp. 29–30.

5. Cecil Murphey, *Keeping My Balance: Spiritual Help When Someone I Love Abuses Drugs* (Louisville, Ky.: Westminster Press, 1988), p. 9.

6. Murphey, *Keeping My Balance*, p. 13.

Body Image

15

Disordered Eating Behavior

We name things so we can talk about them. We put labels on conditions that exist among a number of people so we can describe the symptoms of the conditions. We are, as a society, so efficient about naming and describing conditions that we're apt to lose sight of the person behind the label.

The person behind the label also tends to lose sight of his or her individuality or personhood and can't get past the label. Thus, a person with a disordered eating pattern becomes defined, in his or her mind, as an entire person as an anorexic or a bulimic or an overeater.

To determine what a disordered eating pattern is, I must first identify its opposite. I call it an individual, healthy eating pattern. That is, what is right for the individual when eating is in response to hunger, taste, nutrition, and so on, and weight isn't an issue, nor is body image a barrier to living fully.

Therefore, disordered eating is eating, or not eating, for solace, image, stress, fear, loneliness, control, anger, or any of the issues we've discussed in preceding chapters.

Labels categorize the different relationship issues that disordered eaters have with food. However, I've found that when I group all disordered eaters together, the overriding issue is the relationship with the act of eating and all of the irrelevant issues they combine with the act.

Understanding is important, but action is the solution. Action involves gaining strength, making choices, building boundaries, affirm-

We're apt to lose sight of the person behind the label.

Disordered eating is eating, or not eating, for solace, image, stress, fear, loneliness, control, anger.

Action is the solution.

ing the core self, respecting the body image, and identifying the feelings that trigger problem eating and the peaceful feelings that don't.

Anorexia

Jennifer feared to make decisions.

Jennifer was like a gerbil on a wheel: her refusal to eat gave her power and strength in her family because it brought her attention, which in turn reinforced her power and strength. She liked the attention, but it also trapped her. She challenged her parents to make her decisions for her, yet she wanted to make decisions, so she was in conflict. She feared to make her own decisions, to take the risks and reap the rewards associated with them. She used her strength to run away from the responsibility, and as a consequence, she paralyzed herself.

She needed to work on trusting her core self to handle her problems. She had to trust that her body image didn't need to be perfect, nor did she have to make great accomplishments to succeed. She only had to take risks and assume responsibility for them and know she could trust her choices.

She identified the feelings of fear that occurred when she ate and disempowered them.

Since her core self shrank as she starved herself, that very core self needed affirmation. Once she claimed her core self, she no longer felt empty. By identifying her feelings at the moment that she felt empty, she unmasked them and disarmed them. Then she identified the feelings of fear that occurred when she ate and disempowered them.

Formerly, she used her strength to escape what she feared; now she

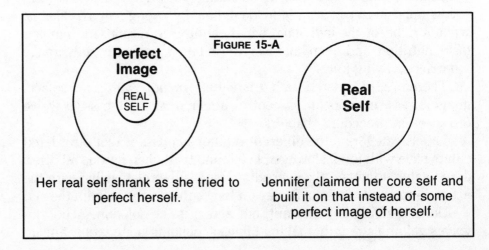

FIGURE 15-A

Perfect Image

REAL SELF

Real Self

Her real self shrank as she tried to perfect herself.

Jennifer claimed her core self and built it on that instead of some perfect image of herself.

is using that strength and building on it. She is claiming her core self, and she no longer feels empty. (See 15-A.)

Bulimia

Food carried the burden of Cindy's bad feelings, so she ate. The purging that followed the bingeing served several purposes. By feeding her bad feelings, the food became the feelings and left her when she vomited. By purging, she escaped responsibility for her feelings and the food, all at once. She also hated her body image, so she punished it by purging the food that her body needed to survive and thus escaped the necessity for taking responsibility for her body.

She needed to stop trying to escape responsibility for her actions. When a situation was difficult, she needed to see that no external safety net was necessary. She needed to build her confidence and trust in her abilities to make the right decisions, and then own her success or failure and see that she had the strength necessary.

Cindy needed to build her confidence and trust in her abilities to make the right decisions.

Cindy worked on identifying her feelings before she binged and before she purged. Owning the feelings took away their power to make her react and showed her that she had a choice. She is working on building a good relationship with herself, being responsible for her choices, and putting confidence in her core self rather than running from it, which made her feel empty until she filled it with food.

She is working on building a good relationship with herself.

┌─**NOTE TO MYSELF**──────────────────┐
I will take responsibility for my actions.
└──────────────────────────────────────┘

Compulsive Dieter

Adam seems to have spent his whole life dieting. It's been one diet after another, each one prompted by another event he feels he must prepare for. Dieting, he says with a laugh, is his career.

The problem is that Adam is a totally self-directed person in all areas but eating. There he gives the power of choice to diet number 10, 15, or 20, so he doesn't have to take responsibility for that moment of eating. That takes away from his core self, which causes him to feel

Adam is a totally self-directed person in all areas but eating.

empty, unfocused, angry, and resentful, so he rebels by going on a binge.

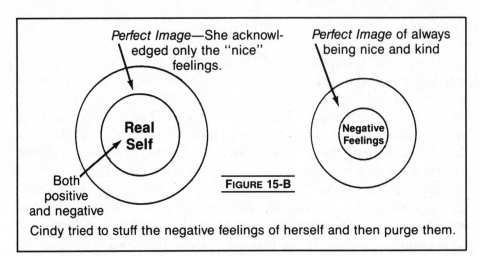

Perfect Image—She acknowledged only the "nice" feelings.

Real Self

Both positive and negative

Perfect Image of always being nice and kind

Negative Feelings

FIGURE 15-B

Cindy tried to stuff the negative feelings of herself and then purge them.

Once all that reactive freight was off the act of eating, his weight stabilized.

Adam began by identifying the feeling when he was ready to go on another diet and then dealing with the feeling. He discovered, not much to his surprise, that he was unhappy with his body image. Learning to respect his body, from that very moment, helped him take ownership of how he looked, how he ate, and how he felt, and the choices he made that affected those feelings. Once all that reactive freight was off the act of eating, his weight stabilized, and he no longer needed a diet plan; he was respectful of his own choices, his own diet.

┌─ **NOTE TO MYSELF** ─────────────────┐
  I will respect my body when I eat.
└──────────────────────────────────────┘

You will lose weight with Inner Eating . . . and it will stay off.

With a diet, you're following an external plan and building no confidence in your powers of choice and decision.

Many compulsive dieters want to lose weight and then begin on the Inner Eating process because Inner Eating doesn't offer instant weight loss. You will lose weight with Inner Eating, if that's what you choose, and it will stay off, if that's what you choose.

The difference between the two is that, with a diet, you're following an external plan and building no confidence in your powers of choice and decision. With Inner Eating, you develop your tools and strengths and reach your goal by power of your choice, and you own it; it's yours and there's no fear that you can't stay there.

Compulsive Overeater

Many things can cause overeating. Perhaps there are core-self issues that persons don't want to, or haven't learned to, handle. Or maybe they just love the taste of food and haven't taken charge of the amounts they eat. Americans serve large portions of food habitually, and they may not even be aware that they overeat until something makes them conscious of it. Perhaps you eat limited amounts all day, but then you overeat at dinner. Be aware of influences around you when you overeat, such as family, loneliness, confusion, or boredom. Identify your trigger and then take charge of its impact on you. Next, identify the quiet times when there is no overeating trigger. Your conscious awareness disarms the power of those situations to influence your eating.

Americans serve large portions of food habitually, and they may not even be aware that they overeat until something makes them conscious of it.

It's possible to be angry at your body and punish or reject it by stuffing it. Identify a time when you feel calm and have freedom to eat without anger, chatter, rejection, or guilt. Then learn to accept your body, or at least to respect it without judgment or defiance.

It's possible to be angry at your body and punish or reject it by stuffing it.

Love affects weight. Charles fell in love, and the weight melted off because his core self was filled with love and felt accepted. When the love relationship ended, the weight came back on. He was able to identify his core self and feelings, affirm himself, and take charge of his choices, his body, and his boundaries. Slowly his weight stabilized at his in-love level, and it stayed there because he filled his core with love and acceptance.

Charles fell in love, and the weight melted off. . . . When the love relationship ended, the weight came back on.

Foods and Moods

Foods influence the state of mind and the body, but what works for one person might not work for another. For example, you may come home from work, have a cookie and a can of soda to hold you over to dinner, and feel draggy and grumpy. Another person who eats the same snack might feel energized and happy.

Sugar calms people, decreases alertness, and makes them feel fatigued.

A common belief is that sugar makes people hyper and gives them a lift. Mothers have kept sugar away from their children, fearing it would cause them to be more active than normal. Recent studies (by biochemists Judith and Richard Wurtman of the Massachusetts Institute of Technology) demonstrate that sugar calms people, decreases alertness, and makes them feel fatigued. (It's connected to the serotonin—one of the brain's chemical messengers—level, which can vary from person to person.)

In another study, Dennis Murphy (a psychiatrist at the National Institute of Mental Health) points to the fact that bodies are different and react differently to the same substance—again serotonin—even from one occasion to another.

If you crave a piece of bread with honey or a glass of milk or a piece of meat, your body is telling you that it requires the particular nutrients in that food.

The final arbiter is you. You have to decide for yourself what is right for you—the amounts of food, the kinds of food, the times you eat. Listen to your body signals. If you crave a piece of bread with honey or a glass of milk or a piece of meat, your body is telling you that it requires the particular nutrients in that food. Only you can make that determination. Your body is unique to you.

Addiction/Attraction

The feeling of attraction or addiction comes not from the food but from your feelings.

If you feel drawn to food and call it addiction, I want to point out again that food is not an addictive substance. The feeling of attraction or addiction comes not from the food but from your feelings. To break the bond, identify the feeling of attraction when and where it happens. What are your personal circumstances at that moment?

Ask yourself, Was there ever a time when this food was available to me and I ate only one or a small amount? Acknowledge and affirm that feeling. That will prove to you that the attraction comes from your mind, your feelings, not some chemical component of the food or your body.

Magnetism, or addiction, is a process of decreasing or diminished choices and feels like you have no Start! and Stop! limits. But you do, and you have proved it in the past on one or more occasions.

"I'm addicted to sugar," Diane said. "Once I start eating, I can't stop. If I eat just one piece of candy, I feel a compulsion to keep eating more."

"In a typical week," I said, "is there ever a time when you could have just a bite or two and then stop?"

After considering my question for several seconds, Diane thought of one. "When my husband and I go out to dinner, he orders dessert. I can have one or two bites of his and then stop."

"Then validate yourself as being able to stop after a few bites."

"But if I order a dessert," she said, "I can't stop until I finish every bite."

"But you can stop if the food is on his plate?"

She said, "Yes."

"Then you have the capability within you to stop."

That was a difficult concept for Diane to identify. Because she felt she had no choice, she decided that she must be addicted. As I tried to show her, it's not that certain foods are addictive; it was a matter of *her* attitude and behavior when she ate.

Choices are directly opposed to addiction. Addiction says that you have no choice. Addiction says that you are compulsively forced to eat, and that you have no opportunity to refuse.

Diane identified that she could stop if her husband ordered dessert for himself. It was a small thing perhaps but a beginning for her. Once she could take charge of her eating, she started learning to make choices.

Sexual Abuse

If sexual abuse is part of your background, you may live with an eating problem in some form. Your core self was invaded without your permission, and your eating arises from your efforts to heal that invasion. By identifying your boundaries and claiming your right to make choices, you can reclaim your core self and resolve your eating problem.

Therapists who specialize in the area of sexual abuse tell me that a high percentage of anorexics and bulimics were sexually abused. One therapist said of her clients, "While not all people with eating disorders were sexually molested, almost all people who were sexually assaulted have eating disorders."

In an article entitled "The Secret Issues of Obesity," Dr. Virginia

"Is there ever a time when you could have just a bite or two and then stop?"

Because Diane felt she had no choice, she decided that she must be addicted.

A high percentage of anorexics and bulimics were sexually abused.

Sexual abuse survivors are overrepresented among obese women.

Porcello, Director of Solutions Weight Management Program, discusses obesity in women. She points out that sexual abuse survivors are over-represented among obese women. She links abuse and obesity:

> Compulsive eating frequently begins soon after sexual abuse occurs, and if women were already prone to turn to food to cope with hard-to-handle feelings, their eating problems worsen. In addition, the dates women begin their first of many, many diets often coincide with the time of their traumatic sexual experiences. And common reactions to sexual abuse—guilt, poor self-esteem, distorted body image, anxiety and a sense of powerlessness, to name a few—are virtually identical to those long associated with obesity and eating problems.
>
> The true tragedy of this situation is that obese, overweight and diet-obsessed women who are also sexual abuse victims are almost always completely unaware of the connection. They believe that fat is the real problem that causes any other problems they might have and that losing weight is the ultimate solution which will remove all obstacles from their path.[1]

Ellen Bass and Laura Davis in their popular book *Courage to Heal* speak less authoritatively:

> Eating difficulties often result from abuse. Young girls who were sexually abused sometimes develop anorexia and bulimia. In a rigidly controlled family system where the abuse is hidden and all appearances are normal, anorexia or bulimia can be a cry for help. For girls who've been pressured into sex they don't want, growing into a woman's body can be terrifying. Anorexia and bulimia can be an attempt to say no, to assert control over their changing bodies.
>
> Compulsive overeating is another way of coping. Survivors may feel that being large will keep them from having to deal with sexual advances.[2]

"Survivors may feel that being large will keep them from having to deal with sexual advances."

Wendy Maltz and Beverly Holman write,

> The development of an eating disorder that results in extreme thinness or in an overweight condition may be an unconscious reaction to . . . incest and a way of avoiding the acceptance of sexual maturity in young adulthood. . . . Overeating can also produce a body that is less attractive and thus less vulnerable to sexual interests of others.

"Overeating can also produce a body that is less attractive and thus less vulnerable to sexual interests of others."

While serving as a protective function for survivors, these extreme conditions seriously jeopardize health and reinforce feelings of social isolation, rejection, and inadequacy. A large number of people suffering from eating disorders were victims of incest.[3]

Survivors of sexual abuse don't simply outgrow their problem; they refocus and shift it to other directions. Having eating disorders is one direction they take. A female who has been victimized by incest or sexual assault wasn't given permission to choose. (These eating disorders occur primarily in women.)

A female who has been victimized by incest or sexual assault wasn't given permission to choose.

"I never felt my body belonged to me," said one such survivor. "My father stole it from me. Is it any wonder that I hated my body?"

This twenty-seven-year-old had no pleasure in her body. She believed her body had been invaded; therefore, she found it disgusting. She wore clothes and hairstyles that made her look unattractive and unappealing to men. Almost from the time the abuse began, she has been overweight. She said, "I thought it would stop anybody getting too close."

An anorexic survivor of abuse usually tries to starve her despised body into nothing. Since her body disgusts her, why would she lavish care on it? That also means she won't provide her body with sufficient nourishment. Because of her trauma, the abused anorexic hasn't had the opportunity to develop a healthy attitude toward herself, much less toward food.

Because of her trauma, the abused anorexic hasn't had the opportunity to develop a healthy attitude toward herself, much less toward food.

"Part of my self was taken from me," said another survivor. "Now I'm trying to reclaim it."

Dr. Henry Cloud discusses crossed boundaries in *When Your World Makes No Sense* and says,

The most basic boundary is the body. . . . When you possess your body, you know that it belongs to you. You can feel it, you can own the pleasure that it brings you through your senses, and you are basically in touch with it. To be out of touch with one's body causes all sorts of problems spiritually, emotionally, and psychologically.

When people have had their bodily boundaries invaded by abuse or control, they may disown them in some way. They learn that their bodies, in a sense, do not belong to them; they belong to others. This is most often true with people who have been sexually abused or mistreated, even as adults.

To invade another person's body boundaries is the most basic act of abuse.[4]

—————————————————— ☐ ——————————————————

If you feel the need for professional help, I hope you'll allow yourself to get it.

If you're a survivor of sexual assault, you may need therapy. If you feel the need for professional help, I hope you'll allow yourself to get it. Along with national organizations, most metropolitan communities have a number of mutual help groups. (At the end of this chapter I've included the names, addresses, and telephone numbers of national organizations.)

Give yourself permission to care for your body.

Whatever method you take to get help, give yourself permission to care for your body. Because it is your body, you already have that permission. You also have the right to be angry with the person who took away your sense of self and body.

You were victimized. But you are a survivor.

One of the most common problems I encounter with survivors is that they assume responsibility for the abuse. "It must have been something I did. For a long time I wouldn't get help because I thought it was my fault," said one woman who was abused by an older brother for two years.

Don't blame yourself for being abused.

Please don't blame yourself for being abused. Remember, you had no choice then because someone else took away your power over your body. But now you are in charge. You couldn't say no then, but you can now. *For your sake,* you need to get past your pain and develop a healthy attitude toward your body.

After a year's therapy, one twenty-two-year-old woman said, "For the first time in my life, my body could say no."

CHAPTER SUMMARY

Labels help us talk about things but limit persons we label. Disordered eating patterns are the opposite of eating in response to hunger, choice, taste, nutrition, and so on. Weight and body image aren't issues. The common issue of disordered eating patterns is the act of eating combined with irrelevant issues. The solution is action. *Anorexia:* Jennifer gave power to food, hated her body image, and feared her decisions. She had to strengthen her core self and trust herself to make choices and identify her fears. *Bulimia:* Cindy used food to carry and purge her of bad feelings. She needed to take responsibility for her feelings, identify them before her binges, and own them. *Compulsive dieter:* Adam was a career dieter, usually before an event, but then he'd gain again. He disliked his body image and needed to respect his body and take ownership of his choices to build confidence. *Compulsive overeater:* Overeating has various causes. Be aware of triggers of overeating and nonovereating times. Emotions can cause overeating. *Foods and moods:* Foods affect individuals differently. *Addiction/ attraction:* Food magnetism comes from feelings, not substance addiction. *Sexual abuse:* Sexual abuse can trigger disordered eating patterns in an effort to replace violated boundaries.

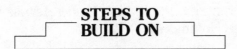

STEPS TO BUILD ON

1. Identify your pattern of disordered eating, if any.

2. Identify the situation in which it happens and the feelings that accompany it. Then use the process of elimination—the grid—to split the emotion from the act of eating.

3. If you feel therapy is called for, please seek it.

4. Affirm your ability to reclaim your healthy act of eating.

National Organizations

Adults Molested as Children United, P.O. Box 952, San Jose, CA 95108, 408-280-5055, focuses on treatment and guided mutual-help groups.

Incest Recovery Association, 6200 North Central Expressway, Suite 209, Dallas, TX 75206, 214-373-6607, is engaged in incest recovery and education.

Incest Resources, Inc., Cambridge Women's Center, 46 Pleasant Street, Cambridge, MA 02139, 617-354-8807, is a nonprofit organization that provides educational and resource material for survivors.

Incest Survivors Resource Network International, P.O. Box 911, Hicksville, NY 11802, 516-935-3031, offers educational resources.

National Coalition Against Sexual Assault (NCASA), 8787 State Street, East St. Louis, IL 62203, 618-398-7764, is a coalition of professionals who provide services for all victims of violence.

PLEA (Prevention, Leadership, Education, Assistance), Box 22, Zia Road, Santa Fe, NM 87505, 505-982-9184, addresses itself primarily to concerns of nonoffending male incest survivors.

The Safer Society Program, Shoreham Depot Road, RR1, Box 24-B, Ortwell, VT 05760, 802-897-7541, is a national project of the New York State Council of Churches, which maintains national lists of agencies, institutions, and individuals providing specialized assessment and treatment for youthful and adult sexual victims and offenders.

Survivors of Childhood Abuse Program (SCAP), 1345 El Centro Avenue, P.O. Box 630, Hollywood, CA 90028, SCAP works on behalf of survivors of incestuous and other dysfunctional family systems. It provides crisis intervention, information, and referrals through the National Child Abuse Hotline, 1-800-422-4453.

NOTES

1. Virginia Porcello, "The Secret Issues of Obesity," *The Jewish Press,* December 30, 1988, p. 49.

2. Ellen Bass and Laura Davis, *Courage to Heal* (New York: Harper and Row, 1988), p. 50.

3. Wendy Maltz and Beverly Holman, *Incest and Sexuality* (Lexington, Mass.: Lexington Books, D. C. Heath & Co., 1987), p. 48.

4. Henry Cloud, *When Your World Makes No Sense* (Nashville: Oliver-Nelson Books, 1990), pp. 134–35.

16

I Wish I Looked Like . . .

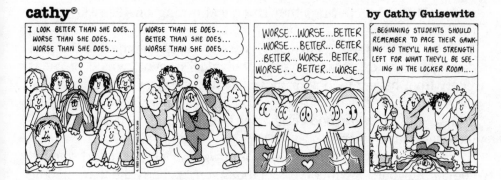

cathy®   **by Cathy Guisewite**

The Cathy character suffers from body-type obsession. This clinical term refers to the preoccupation with a distorted view of one's body image. Body-type obsessives are preoccupied with becoming and remaining skinny or muscular or whatever their ideal form may be.

If body-type obsession stayed only in the mind, it might not be a serious problem. However, as people become fixated on attaining a perfect body, they become irritable, listless, and moody, all classic symptoms of depression. Their preoccupation with body image interferes with the rest of their lives. Research indicates that these people often set themselves up in situations where they will probably fail,

Body-type obsessives are preoccupied with becoming and remaining skinny or muscular or whatever their ideal form may be.

which only increases their depressed feelings and makes them look more longingly at the physical image they can't have.

The healthy flip side is body awareness, which means being aware of your body and its limitations for such things as size and muscle development. You take charge of your body when you look at it realistically and accept it as it is now. Then you commit yourself to do your best for your body and give it loving care. A major goal of Inner Eating is to teach you body awareness and to help you accept that, though body types differ, each one is perfectly valid and deserves to be healthy and respected.

You take charge of your body when you look at it realistically and accept it as it is now.

The biggest obstacle to overcome in body awareness is body comparison. I don't want you to be like poor Cathy, who was so caught up in thinking about how others look and wishing she was like them that she couldn't do anything productive for herself.

By contrast, in my exercise classes I focus on each individual student because each one is important. During the exercises, they're seldom aware of what goes on around them because they're not competing or comparing; they're concentrating on themselves, on their own bodies.

They're not competing or comparing; they're concentrating on themselves, on their own bodies.

Most of the time the participants are working on different things. I create specific exercises for each individual's needs, which provides safety from having to look or move like anyone else. Each person can think, *It's okay. I'm safe here. I don't have to worry about doing an exercise as well as anybody else.* Each body is self-owned and responsible only to its owner!

If you don't own your body as it is now, invariably you find yourself comparing yourself with others. "I thought everybody did that," people tell me.

A fundamental definition of comparison is contrasting two things on a better-worse, superior-inferior scale. Usually people consider their own bodies losers in the contest. Losing the contest damages the ego and often affects the eating pattern. Compulsive eaters constantly compare themselves with thinner individuals. They may react by saying, "That person is thin, so I'll watch how she eats, do the same thing, and then get thin, too." Or they may reverse it by comparing their eating with that of people heavier than they are: "How can he stay so fat and eat so little?"

Compulsive eaters constantly compare themselves with thinner individuals.

When individuals compare the amounts they eat with the amounts of others, I point out four things.

1. You see only the other's public eating.
2. Most indulging is done in secret.
3. Comparing doesn't help your sense of self-worth.
4. You have to discover your eating needs; you don't eat successfully by following another's plan or program (like the diet mentality).

Imitating another's eating might help you experiment with other eating models, but you need to find your own pattern because bodies, appetites, and metabolisms differ. Each person needs to find his or her own pattern. Some people are hungry when they first get up; others don't feel hunger for an hour or two afterward. Some people do well on three meals; others, six. Some are natural grazers, but their total food intake may still be less than those with set meals.

Each person needs to find his or her own pattern.

It's the same with comparing bodies. If your friend, who is twenty-five pounds overweight, goes on a diet and loses weight, you say to yourself, *It must work, so I'll do the same thing. Then I can look like my friend.*

Comparisons sabotage you. You may start out feeling good in an exercise program, but when you pause to glance at the person near you, what happens? You start comparing: *She's thinner. I'd better go on a diet.* Or you may think, *He's in good shape. Sure wish I had that body. Maybe I can find out what he does to get in shape like that.* It's a game you can't win. Even if you scrupulously follow another's regimen, you won't achieve a similar body because each person is unique. Inevitably you come out feeling inferior because you'll always find someone who's closer to your ideal image than you are.

Even if you scrupulously follow another's regimen, you won't achieve a similar body because each person is unique.

Here are typical reactions clients have shared with me, and I've been through some of them myself.

- "I'm jealous of her body."
- "Looking at him makes me angry. He doesn't seem to do anything special, and he looks like that. Why do I have to have the weight problem?"
- "She's thin. She's probably conceited."
- "How can I get to look like that?"
- "I would be happy if I didn't have this weight dragging me down all the time."

I know women who cut out pictures of models and stick them on the refrigerator. Their goal is to look like the photos. They'll say to themselves, "That's how I want to be. That's what I'm going to look like." They eat and exercise and try to match the image. After a few days, or maybe weeks, they look in their mirrors and see that they're not matching up, most likely because they are a different body type altogether. Discouraged, they're likely to go into an erratic eating pattern of gobbling or dieting. Either way they lose the comparison game.

---NOTE TO MYSELF---

I don't have to be perfect; I only have to be me.

Before I learned to own my body, I compared myself with others, a test I usually failed. Then a few years ago I noticed that I had stopped; I no longer felt the need to be like anyone but me.

---NOTE TO MYSELF---

Self-acceptance makes me stronger every day.

It isn't easy to change habits, but you can do it.

If you do the comparison number on yourself, you can get away from it, too. It isn't easy to change habits, but you can do it. In my classes, I notice that newcomers start comparing automatically because they're used to doing that. After a while, they change their focus, get in touch with their bodies, and start appreciating their unique anatomies. Comparing then revolves around feeling how different muscles in their bodies work together. My clients realize that they don't have to compare looks and appearances, and they find a new peace and contentment with their goals and bodies.

Those who have been with the program for some time already have excellent figures, come dressed in the finest workout clothes, and strut as if they're giving a performance.

By contrast, several clients have told me about their sad experiences after joining other exercise programs. They say that those who have been with the program for some time already have excellent figures, come dressed in the finest workout clothes, and strut as if they're giving a performance. (True or not, that's the typical beginner's perception of the more advanced exercise programs.) Newcomers and persons still out of shape feel uncomfortable and inferior.

"It's like going into a place where everyone there can dance except me," said one woman. "I just feel out of place."

In one of my exercise classes, a large woman listened in amazement to the conversation of the others when they grumbled about being dissatisfied with their bodies. "They looked great to me," she said.

"Suppose a woman larger than you came into this class," I said. "How do you think you'd look to her?"

"Oh, yeah," she said. "I'd look pretty good to her, wouldn't I?"

"If you understand that," I said, "you can move on toward accepting your body. You are you, and you'll never look exactly like anyone else."

The more you work with your muscles, the more you create a sense of ownership. As you feel your stomach muscles, for instance, and learn to tighten and relax them, you begin to own them.

She's beginning to see herself as she really is, a unique and beautiful person.

Just as it was with me, a gradual acceptance happens. I've seen it occur again and again. Even though you realize your body isn't perfect, that doesn't trouble you the way it did before. You become so thrilled with gaining control over your body that you forget about comparing.

---------------------□----------------------

A great deal of work needs to be done in body acceptance. In the late 1980s a *Glamour* magazine survey discovered that 90 percent of the readers disliked their bodies. Add this to a growing list of statistics:

- Americans spent 33 million dollars for diet products in 1989.
- The average woman who seeks the advice of a nutritionist, doctor, or weight-loss clinic to lose weight has already been on six to ten diets, as well as having purchased numerous diet books.
- Thirty-one percent of American women (ages 19–39) told the Gallup Poll that they diet at least once a month.[1]

Although we have less information about men and their body comparisons, the evidence is accumulating that men are becoming more obsessed about their bodies. Within the next decade I expect to see a greater focus on the problems men encounter with their quest for physical perfection.

Men are becoming more obsessed about their bodies.

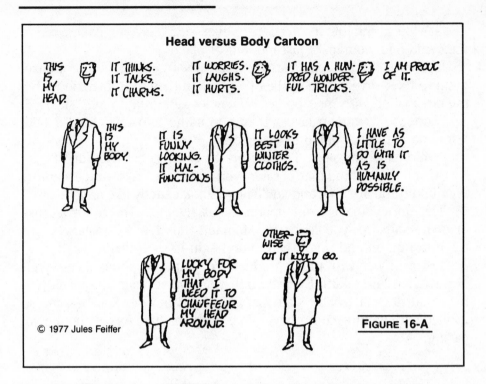

Head versus Body Cartoon

© 1977 Jules Feiffer

FIGURE 16-A

The average man wants to look like Rambo or the Marlboro Man.

According to an article in *American Health,* the average man wants to look like Rambo or the Marlboro Man. Weight itself isn't as important for men as it is for women; they think more in terms of large muscles and broad chests:

> The average man says his shoulders and chest are both medium width, but he'd like each to be broader. He describes himself as lean, but would rather be muscular. At the same time, he'd like to be an inch taller. And he thinks all these changes would make him more attractive to women. . . . the media help promote the image of men as tough, physically strong, competitive and forceful.[2]

I encourage clients to go through their closets and keep only the items they feel good in. If you do, and I hope you will, allow yourself to trust your feelings. Do you like how the garment makes you feel? Maybe you've never thought about it before, but clothes affect your attitude toward yourself.

Clothes affect your attitude toward yourself.

If you're not aware of your responses to texture and color, take note of them for the next week. When you choose a garment consider how it makes you feel—comfortable, sharp, attractive, fun, professional, calm, relaxed, enthusiastic, or competent. Does it make you feel more at home in your body? Feeling at home in your body makes it easier for you to respect it and identify your core self. That will help you claim your unique, smaller zone of eating.

You are you now. When you accept yourself, you like and honor yourself, and you project an aura of likability and calm that is inviting to other people. People are drawn to those who accept themselves.

When you accept your-self, you like and honor yourself.

Maybe you're not Antony or Cleopatra. You're you—unique and beautiful in your special way and a most valuable person.

┌─**NOTE TO MYSELF**──────────────────┐
I will be gentle with myself.
└──────────────────────────────────────┘

Give yourself the gift of a cleared place in your forest of demand. When the sun of self-affirmation and free choice warms your shoulders, you will grow in a new, calm, and peaceful way. Then, when people compliment you on your sense of self-possession and serenity, you can answer in all honesty, "Thank you."

CHAPTER SUMMARY

Body-type obsession causes unfavorable comparisons with others. Body awareness accepts the body as it is now. Each body is unique and has its specific needs and strengths, so modeling yourself on another's image can be destructive. Review your wardrobe for clothes that make you feel good when you wear them. You are special, unique, and valuable—now.

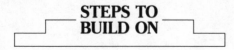

**STEPS TO
BUILD ON**

1. Throw out your diet-incentive pictures.
2. Weed out your wardrobe for clothes that don't encourage you to feel good.

3. Imagine yourself free from all self-judgmental comparison, and allow the image to come true.

4. Honor yourself.

5. Accept compliments without denial, honoring the giver's perception that a compliment is due.

NOTES

1. Kelly Brownell, "The Yo-Yo Trap," *American Health,* March 1988, p. 78.

2. A. G. Britton, "Make Friends with Your Body," *American Health,* July-August 1988, p. 71.

17

Reclaiming Your Body

Now that you've stopped comparing your body type with others, let's consider the kind of body you have, so you can see more clearly that yours is unlike any other.

"My weight is a problem," she said. "I'm still ten pounds too heavy." Most people would have considered Marcia perfect for her size. She was five five, weighed 120, and was obsessed about losing more weight.

I knew I had to help her see that her weight wasn't the problem; she wasn't aware of her body's limitations within her body type. She was a mesomorph, which is a muscular type and unlikely to be rail thin.

Like Marcia, your image of your body helps you determine how you see yourself as a total person. I believe that the body is good; it is a basic part of who you are. Part of self-caring is caring for the body. And your body is different from anyone else's. It concerns me that most exercise programs try to fit everybody, never seeming to consider various body types. People do come in all shapes and sizes, and they're all valid.

You were born with a particular type of body because of genetic factors. You can't do much to change your type, but you can accept it and treat it lovingly.

Half a century ago, researchers at Columbia University began the first modern typing of the human body. Commonly we divide human

She was five five, weighed 120, and was obsessed about losing more weight.

Most exercise programs try to fit everybody, never seeming to consider various body types.

Commonly we divide human bodies into three basic types.

bodies into three basic types. The classic definitions refer to the extremes. If you are like most people, you're a combination of these types:

the ectomorph,
the endomorph, and
the mesomorph.

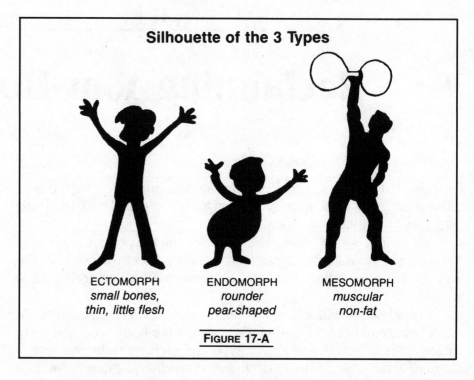

Silhouette of the 3 Types

ECTOMORPH
*small bones,
thin, little flesh*

ENDOMORPH
*rounder
pear-shaped*

MESOMORPH
*muscular
non-fat*

FIGURE 17-A

If you're an ectomorph, you have little flesh to cover small bones, and you're thin. If you're an endomorph, you have an inherited tendency to be rounder and more pear-shaped. Or if you're a mesomorph, you have a thicker, muscular build with solid flesh but are relatively free of excess fat.

In the article, "Quest for the Best," the author states clearly what we can and cannot change:

> Despite a decade of being told we are each masters of our own bodies, there are certain things that can't be changed. The starting point for body shape is, after all, bone structure. Certain body areas,

"Certain body areas, especially shoulders and hips—are as or more dependent on bone than fat or muscle for their shape."

especially shoulders and hips—are as or more dependent on bone than fat or muscle for their shape. Diet and exercise can increase bone density, the amount of calcium stored within bone tissue, but there's nothing that can be done to change the body frame that bones provide.[1]

When you care for your body and learn what's best for it, you learn its limits and the changes possible. Whatever your body type, this is the given with which you live. (See 17-A.) An important step in accepting yourself is understanding your body type and owning it, then setting boundaries for it.

You may gauge your self-worth by the shape of your body or the numbers on your bathroom scale. If you do, I hope you'll move away from that kind of illusory thinking because it's self-destructive.

Your perception of yourself also plays a significant role in what you're willing to do for your body. If you think of yourself as hopelessly fat, you're not likely to take much interest in your body. Yet your body is your outer aspect and, therefore, part of your expression of life.

If you think of yourself as hopelessly fat, you're not likely to take much interest in your body.

Dr. Alexander Lowen, a pioneer in connecting psychoanalytic work with the body, says,

A body is forsaken when it becomes a source of pain and humiliation instead of pleasure and pride. Under these conditions the person refuses to accept or identify with his body. He turns against it. He may ignore it or he may attempt to transform it into a more desirable object by dieting, weight lifting, etc.

The alive body is characterized by a life of its own. It has a motility independent of ego control which is manifested by the spontaneity of its gestures and the vivacity of its expression. It hums, it vibrates, it glows. It is charged with feeling. The first difficulty that one encounters with patients in search of identity is that they are not aware of the lack of aliveness in their bodies. People are so accustomed to thinking of the body as an instrument or a tool of the mind that they accept its relative deadness as a normal state. They measure bodies in pounds and inches and compare their shape with idealized forms, completely ignoring the fact that what is important is how the body feels.[2]

"People are so accustomed to thinking of the body as an instrument or a tool of the mind that they accept its relative deadness as a normal state."

┌─ **NOTE TO MYSELF** ─────────────────────┐
My body is an integral part of ME.
└──┘

Don't minimize the personal importance of the things you do through and with your body.

The way you think and feel about your body expresses itself in the way you think and feel about the world around you and how you respond to that world. You experience the world through your physical senses. The body is more than just an object or a thing. Your physical self is expressed through your body, and it's vital that you don't minimize the personal importance of the things you do through and with your body. When you don't consider your body personal, you diminish your relationships with others. For you, the world becomes foreign, external, and perhaps frightening.

In the article "The Body Has its Reasons," the importance of feeling unity with our bodies is stated again:

> Our body . . . is not opposed to our intelligence, to our feelings, to our souls. It includes them and shelters them. By becoming aware of our body we give ourselves access to our entire being—for body and spirit, mental and physical, and strength and weakness, present not our duality but our unity.[3]

──────────── □ ────────────

Do you ever wonder why we have such a negative view of the body? It goes back to at least 400 B.C., to the philosophies of Plato and Aristotle, who held that the body is inferior to the spirit or soul. They proposed that the body was a union between form and matter. While the mother (*mater,* matter) supplied the raw material—obviously the inferior aspect to these men—the father contributed the soul—the higher form.

St. Paul . . . wrote two thousand years ago that the body is God's temple.

Platonic thought deeply influenced Western perceptions through the present century. Yet, interestingly, St. Paul, who was born in the Greek city of Tarsus, wrote two thousand years ago that the body is God's temple. Only in the past few decades have we begun to embrace that understanding as having insight and value.

Because of the far-reaching effects of Platonic philosophy, you may have grown up thinking of your body as something to be ignored, especially when your body was involved in sexual activity. We are learning now to say that the body is good.

———————————— ☐ ————————————

When I created Inner Eating, I sensed there had to be a process to get people to the point that

- they had less anxiety about the act of eating.
- they could appreciate and value their bodies as sacred vessels.
- they could get past the ideal body image that was blocking them.

Just having a thin body is not the answer. There are people in diet clinics searching for a path to these conclusions. There are people stuck in their lives for lack of this understanding. If they can only un-

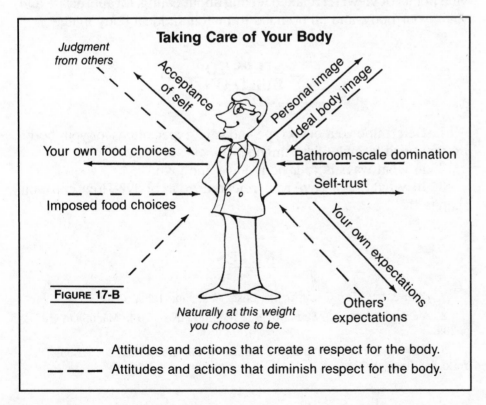

Taking Care of Your Body

Judgment from others

Acceptance of self

Personal image

Ideal body image

Your own food choices

Bathroom-scale domination

Self-trust

Imposed food choices

Your own expectations

Others' expectations

Naturally at this weight you choose to be.

FIGURE 17-B

———— Attitudes and actions that create a respect for the body.

– – – – Attitudes and actions that diminish respect for the body.

derstand and internalize these three crucial concepts, they can end their search and direct their energies more joyfully to taking care of their bodies. (See 17-B.)

┌─ **NOTE TO MYSELF** ─────────────────────┐

I'm going to spend my energy being a more joyful me.

└──┘

CHAPTER SUMMARY

Marcia needed to understand and work with her body type. There are three basic body types: ectomorph, endomorph, and mesomorph. Lowen says that an accepted body is a dynamic body. How you feel about your body influences how you feel about your world. There are three vital points of view: (1) relaxed feeling about eating, (2) appreciate and value your body, and (3) no need to match an ideal body image.

STEPS TO BUILD ON

1. Determine your body type and your expectations for your body. Do you need to make adjustments?

2. In what ways is your body alive and joyful?

3. In what ways have you rejected your body? How can you change that?

NOTES

1. Peter Jaret, "The Quest for the Best," *Self,* June 1989, p. 108.

2. Alexander Lowen, *The Betrayal of the Body* (New York: Macmillan, 1967), p. 209.

3. Therese Bertherat and Carol Bernstein, *The Body Has Its Reasons* (New York: Pantheon, 1977).

18

Fine-Tuning Your Body

To neglect one's body for any other advantage in life is the greatest of follies.—Arthur Schopenhauer

It is the mind itself which shapes the body.—Friedrich von Schiller

Physical fitness has been important to me as long as I can remember. In college I majored in physical education and health, and then I taught at Westwood Junior High in the St. Louis Park schools, a suburb of Minneapolis. My love of health and fitness grew when I teamed up with fellow teachers Betty Litten and Marge Mathews. We truly enjoyed teaching and creating activities that were both fun and healthy for the students.

We put exercises to music long before the terms *aerobic dance* and *Jazzercize* became known across the country. We had fun with movement, and we wanted to pass the feeling on to our students.

We had fun with movement, and we wanted to pass the feeling on.

As I started a family, my interest in caring for the body intensified. I taught in various exercise programs, and continued to learn about fitness. I concentrated on staying in tune with my body, identifying my eating pattern, and getting away from external messages about what I should eat and how I should look.

While I was developing my concepts, I took a course from an organization that specialized in teaching corrective exercises to people who had done improper movement and damaged their bodies. I read a great deal, kept up with all the research, and held exercise classes in my home. By working with a small number of people, I believed I could get more in touch with how my students were feeling about their bodies. And I learned.

With all of that background and the freedom to have my own studio, I could teach, learn, grow, and pass on what I learned to my students. I wanted them to own their bodies and their eating, and not match some image. When I established the Fitness Forum (a home-based exercise-and-eating consultancy) in 1980, I felt I was moving in the right direction. The combination of proper exercise and healthy eating patterns led to a positive body image.

The combination of proper exercise and healthy eating patterns led to a positive body image.

In addition to making you feel and look better, getting in good physical shape through a sensible exercise program has a wide range of benefits, including:

- speeding up the metabolism
- reducing the percentage of body fat
- strengthening the heart
- making the muscles more efficient
- improving posture

To maximize these benefits, I created a general program that I adjusted according to each individual's needs.

Before starting a program, respect your body by getting a complete physical.

However, before starting a program, respect your body by getting a complete physical. You can't see what is going on in your body; only tests can give you that information. With our advanced medical knowledge, there's so much we can prevent and heal if we just stay knowledgeable as to what is going on with our bodies. Listening to your body and knowing what's going on inside are essential to preventative medicine.

I don't stand in front of my exercise classes and have everyone imitate what I'm doing. I move among the students, working with them individually, showing them the movements, and teaching them how to listen to their bodies. If they have an injury, I show them how to work around it. If their abdominal muscles are weaker than their leg muscles, I'll pull them off some leg exercises and have them concentrate more on the abdominals.

I'm constantly showing them how to feel the muscles they're trying to tone by having them move into different positions to get the full benefit of the exercise.

They often hear me say, "When you exercise, listen to your body. It's not *what* you do but *how* you do it that counts."

[I haven't included here the specific exercises I do in my classes—that would take another book. You can get a number of good books on exercise from a bookstore or library. These books I highly recommend: *Callanetics* and *Callanetics for the Back* by Callan Pinckney; *The Pilates Method of Physical and Mental Conditioning* by Philip Friedman and Gail Eisen; *Awake! Aware! Alive!: Exercises for a Vital Body* by Lydia Bach (the Lotte Berk Method); *The Alexander Technique* by Judith Leibowitz and Bill Connington; *Fit or Fat* by Covert Bailey; and *Stretching* by Bob Anderson.]

I want to discuss four basic components of a complete exercise program and give a brief discussion as to what to look for. As in nutrition, there are a few basic things you need to know and from then on you listen to your body.

The four basic components are *endurance* (aerobics), *strength* (strong stomach muscles; tightened buttocks muscles; upper body strength; strong leg muscles), *flexibility,* and *posture.*

Endurance

Your heart is a muscle. It needs exercise just like every other muscle in your body. Without exercise, you may get out of breath walking up a flight of stairs or have a heart attack running for that tennis shot you used to reach. The heart is the most important muscle to exercise—it sustains your life! But how do you exercise it? Through aerobic exercise. There are so many different and creative ways to get aerobic exercise—cycling, walking, jogging, swimming, rollerskating, rollerblading, cross-country skiing, ice skating, rope jumping, dancing, stepping (the new exercise in health clubs), rowing, or just running in place. You can exercise inside or outside, with equipment or without equipment, in fancy exercise wear or just sweats. And how long is considered enough by the American College of Sports Medicine? At least three twenty-minute workouts a week that sustain a target heart rate of at least 60 percent of maximum. In my classes, I'll have my clients check their heart rate periodically during the twenty-minute

"It's not what you do but how you do it that counts."

You can get a number of good books on exercise from a bookstore or library.

The heart is the most important muscle to exercise—it sustains your life!

aerobic workout. For six seconds, they stop and check their pulse rates and then multiply by 10 to get beats per minute. Then they determine if they are at least 60 to 80 percent of their maximum heart rate based on their age. They adjust their activity accordingly.

Now sixty minutes per week (based on three twenty-minute sessions per week) doesn't seem like a lot of time to spend to keep your most important muscle in your body in shape. Yet comments that appeared in *Fitness Without Exercise,* tell us something different:

> Despite what the athletic shoe and yogurt commercials would have us believe, only 10 to 15 percent of U.S. adults currently do enough exercise (at least three twenty-minute workouts a week that sustain a target heart rate of at least 60 percent of maximum) to qualify as aerobically fit according to standards set by the American College of Sports Medicine (ACSM). The rest of us either have attempted a fitness program and failed, or we have chosen simply to ignore the fitness call entirely.[1]

Exercise is fun! It's movement! If it isn't fun, don't do it.

Perhaps the "call to fitness" has been so organized, advertised, equipped, and analyzed that we've lost the joy of it. Exercise is fun! It's movement! If it isn't fun, don't do it. Find something else that is fun for you, tones your muscles, and exercises your heart. Choose your own exercise path, but choose it!

Run on the beach, skip down a hill, ride a bike, play with your children, but play.

If you've lost the joy of movement—something called exercise— you may avoid it because it's work, and you probably make excuses like those in 18-A. If that's so, find what's fun for you and recapture the joy of movement you had as a child. Run on the beach, skip down a hill, ride a bike, play with your children, but play.

┌─ **NOTE TO MYSELF** ──────────────────────────┐
  I will play for the joy of it.
└──┘

Strength

Your skeletal structure is wrapped in muscle, which gives your body strength and flexibility. If your body has strength, the muscles will support the joints and the bones. There are many different exer-

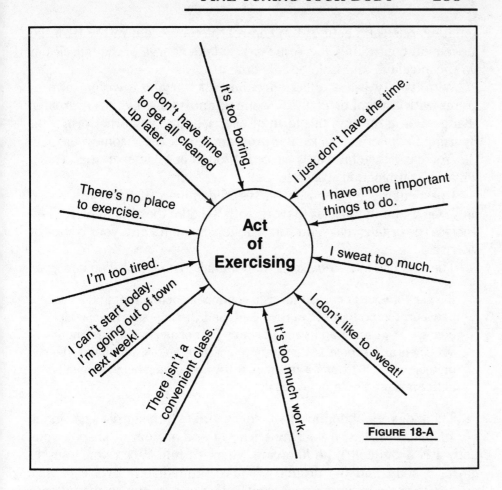

I don't have time
to get all cleaned
up later.

It's too boring.

I just don't have the time.

I have more important
things to do.

There's no place
to exercise.

**Act
of
Exercising**

I'm too tired.

I sweat too much.

I can't start today.
I'm going out of town
next week!

There isn't a
convenient class.

It's too much work.

I don't like to sweat!

FIGURE 18-A

cises that will add strength to your body. Using weight machines, rubber bands, or just your own body are just a few. Proceed with caution, but *do* proceed!

Many exercise programs in gyms, in health spas, and especially on TV will encourage you to kick your legs and do strenuous exercises—but they don't teach you how to get in touch with your body. Some programs also fail to realize or point out that each body is unique. They function much like diet programs in that they give external boundaries and imply that all bodies are the same.

One exception is Callanetics. If you want to buy an exercise video, I highly recommend *Callanetics,* or you might also be interested in Callan Pinckney's best-selling book by the same title.

Pinckney's statement about her exercises parallels my philosophy about exercise and eating: You control the movement rather than the movement controlling you. You learn to take charge of the muscles in slow, controlled, and isolated movements.

You can't tone fat. Fat is burned through aerobic exercises.

With twenty years' experience, and after trying a variety of programs with a number of men, women, and teens, I've seen greater changes come through this form of exercise than any other program. By using Callanetics or a similar program, you learn to tone your muscle. You can't tone fat. Fat is burned through aerobic exercises. That's why the combination works so well.

I particularly concentrate on the abdominals. If I had to choose only one group of muscles to work with, I'd take the abdominals. They enclose the organs that send your hunger signal. It's also your center of gravity.

The Pilates Method calls the abdominals the *center*. The center is

> the part of your body that forms a continuous bond, front and back, between the bottom of your rib cage and the line across your hip-bones. . . . Firming and strengthening your center while keeping it stretched and supple is the prime physical result of practicing the methods. . . . It means a trimmer waist and flatter belly; it means better posture and a more regal carriage.[2]

When your muscle girdle is snug and fits properly, you're immediately aware of any change in the expand-muscles.

Think of your abdominals as a loose girdle. If the girdle sags and is out of shape (that is, if your muscles sag and are out of shape), your body has a difficult time knowing when it's full. When your muscle girdle is snug and fits properly, you're immediately aware of any change in the expand-muscles. You'll start to experience the fullness from your food more quickly if you have a tight pelvic girdle.

Having tight abdominal muscles is also like wearing snug-fitting jeans. If you eat more and expand your stomach, the pressure from those jeans give you a choice: stop eating or loosen your jeans, because the tightness feels uncomfortable. Toned muscles send you clearer messages when the stomach is full.

Strong abdominal muscles working with the back muscles can improve performance in any sport and make you look more graceful and attractive all the time. But when you don't pay attention to your abdominal muscles and keep them in shape, here are the tendencies:

- Your stomach sags forward.
- Your lower back sags.

- Your head hangs forward.
- Your lower back muscles ache because they do too much work.

Your tendency will probably be to push the muscle out when you do sit-ups. I don't teach my clients to do full sit-ups, but partial sit-ups called abdominal crunches with knees bent. The crunch uses all of the abdominal muscles. But don't be misled into thinking that just doing abdominal crunches will flatten your stomach. They are the only muscles that you can tighten either by pulling them in or by letting them out. If you push them out, you'll get a larger stomach (although quite a firm one) instead of a smaller one. Because you're exercising the muscles by pushing them out, you're creating what I call a toned pot. I say, "When doing exercises, train the way you want the muscle to look. You'll want to learn to walk around with your abdominal muscles pulled in, so pull them in while you do sit-ups."

"When doing exercises, train the way you want the muscle to look. You'll want to learn to walk around with your stomach muscle pulled in, so pull it in while you do abdominal crunches."

Flexibility

Flexibility means limberness and pliability. Flexibility guards against pulled or torn muscles and affects the quality of your life. Good flexibility springs from the spine, primarily from the body's two key compensatory curves at the head and neck, and from the lower back and pelvis. A limber body moves easily and assuredly with muscles and connective tissues strong and stretched.

Remember when you are stretching your muscles to move into the stretch slowly, feel the muscle stretch, and hold that position, preferably for fifteen to twenty seconds. Don't bounce—just hold. If you can't hold the stretch because it hurts, you have gone too far. Back off! Make it a stretch not a strain. Every muscle that is strengthened with an exercise need also be stretched for flexibility. Strength and flexibility will tone a muscle nicely.

Posture

I work a lot with posture and show people how to align the body. When I analyze people's posture, I observe them from the side. I look for a straight line with four parts of their body aligned: ear lobe, shoulder, hip, and ankle.

When the four points are in straight line, the person has good posture. If they have poor posture, I will add specific exercises that will correct this. Good posture results from engaging the abdominal muscles so your body starts naturally to align itself. With toned muscles, your posture becomes better because you have the muscle structure to support the bones that allow you to stand tall.

Some people tend to lean forward. The head goes first, and the body trails behind. If this describes you, you may be trying to leave the body behind symbolically. You may be indicating that you dislike your body. Or maybe you're in such a compulsive rush that your body can't keep up.

While we do the exercises, I check posture to see how the body is aligned during the movement. I check the line-up of the knees, tension in the shoulders, and position of the lower back.

Knees over toes. When doing any exercise, the knees will have more support if you keep them lined up with the toes. Some experts hang a string from the middle of the kneecap. If you're moving correctly, it will fall over the second or third toe. If the ankle turns outward, the string is beside the foot. Aside from the fact that ankles turned outward don't look as attractive, the knees get a nasty twist every time the joint bends.

Shoulders. Someone has said that many people wear their shoulders as if they were earrings. The shoulders have crept up to the earlobes and can cause cramps, muscle problems, and even pinched nerve pain.

Drop your shoulders without tensing your muscles to push them down.

If you're having tension there, lift your shoulders and then let them drop gently and naturally into place. Any time you become aware of them creeping upward, just drop them without tensing your muscles to push them down. Relax the upper body, especially the chest, and allow your shoulders to fall into place.

The back. I concentrate on correct movement because my philosophy centers on prevention. Good posture and strong stomach muscles will go a long way toward preventing back problems.

Think of good posture that keeps the spine in line.

Instead of a rigid-straight back, a relaxed, aligned spine has curves that help it spring back. Forget the old military command "Suck in that chin! Pull in that gut! Throw back those shoulders!" Instead, think of good posture that keeps the spine in line. This includes

- strong abdominal muscles,
- knees aligned,
- joints slightly soft (not locked),
- shoulders down and relaxed, and
- head up.

┌─**NOTE TO MYSELF**────────────────┐
│   *I will keep my spine aligned.*   │
└──────────────────────────────────┘

With the four components (endurance, strength, flexibility, and posture) in mind, commit yourself to a good fitness program. Whatever program you undertake, here are three simple reminders:

- You're not doing this for performance.
- You're not doing this to see how many repetitions you can complete.
- You are learning to *feel* each muscle you're working with.

In my exercise classes, I often say, "Tighten the muscle."
"Am I tightening it?" a newcomer will ask.
"Do you feel yourself tightening the muscle?"
"I don't know. How do I tell?"
That's not an unusual answer. Some people are so disconnected from their bodies, they have no idea how to tighten a muscle. They've allowed the body to exist as a disconnected entity from themselves. I especially like *Callanetics* because the exercises have as much to do with the mind as with the body. The mind has to cooperate in telling you to tighten the muscle.
When someone still doesn't know if he or she is tightening, I touch that particular muscle. "Here, this one. Tighten it." That's usually all it takes to follow my instructions.

Some people are so disconnected from their bodies, they have no idea how to tighten a muscle.

Four of my clients will give you some idea of individual differences.

1. *Sharon Dudziak* had never done any exercise before and had never participated in sports; she was frustrated the first few sessions. Because she was out of touch with her body, it took her a long time to build up endurance. Gradually she felt the benefit and no longer became exhausted after walking up a flight of stairs.

Sharon has a success story because she stayed with the program. She now understands what to do with the muscles—and she does it.

2. *Mary Pagnucco* had been a dancer—which would imply she was connected with her body. The first time she came for exercises, I said, "Mary, tighten the lower part of the buttock muscles."

"How do I do that?"

That answer caught me by surprise. As I learned from Mary, and later from others, she had a talent for dancing and she moved correctly; however, it was a matter of doing steps and motions, not understanding her body.

3. *Susie Wilson* is an avid cross-country skier and golfer. She excels in any sport she tries. Yet she also had little connection with her body. It took her a month to learn to work correctly her abdominal muscles. Although she was active in sports, Susie's body had areas of weak muscle tone.

In the last few years an interesting thing has happened. When people first attend my exercise classes, they ask, "Why can't I get to that muscle? Why can't my brain connect to the muscle?"

"Don't worry about it," one of the other students will say before I can answer. "Stay with it. Eventually it'll connect. It did with me."

4. *Chris,* who couldn't engage her abdominal muscles, insisted, "Listen, Shirley, I can't do it. There just aren't any muscles in my stomach."

"You have them. You'll soon learn to feel your muscles."

"Not in my stomach."

"Yes," I insisted, "in your stomach."

She didn't believe me. But later she squealed, "I felt it! There is something there!"

Once people have that first experience, they know what it feels like to be in touch with a part of the body. From then on they can engage and disengage muscles. They know that since they can take charge of that muscle, eventually they can master the whole body.

"Tighten the lower part of the buttock muscles." "How do I do that?"

"I can't do it. There just aren't any muscles in my stomach."

Later she squealed, "I felt it! There is something there!"

Think of your body as a miracle machine. Daily you receive all kinds of coded messages ranging from hunger to satisfaction, from pain to tiredness. Unfortunately, like most other people, you probably haven't been listening. By not listening, you have cut off the messages. One reason for this nonhearing is that the media have paraded pictures of gorgeous bodies before you—all of them quite different from yours. You probably got caught in trying to fit that image or hated your body because you realized you couldn't. I hope you'll learn to be in touch with your body, respect it as it is, and enjoy it.

Daily you receive all kinds of coded messages ranging from hunger to satisfaction, from pain to tiredness.

> ┌─ **NOTE TO MYSELF** ─────────────
> *I am where I'm supposed to be. From this spot I can grow.*

Work with who you are and what you have. You not only have a body but you are a body; it's not just something that joins you at the neck. A friend of mine daily prays, "Dear God, thank You for making me a unique, unrepeatable miracle."

"Dear God, thank You for making me a unique, unrepeatable miracle."

As you learn to listen to your body, you'll recognize the difference between a tightened muscle and a relaxed one. If you are under stress—at home or at work—you'll be able to feel your muscles starting to tighten. Your body is saying, "Do something for me. If you don't, I'll get tighter and tighter." You'll know what to do to relax that stressed muscle. When stress creeps into your shoulders at work, you'll be able to say, "Now I know where I put stress in my body because I can feel my body tightening up there."

As you tone up, you also learn to trust the feelings of your body. Your body is wiser than you may think and constantly gives you messages about yourself. For instance, your body tells you when you're

Your body is wiser than you may think and constantly gives you messages about yourself.

- tired,
- ill,

- overworked,
- sleepy,
- out of shape,
- anxious,
- hungry, or
- full.

You have to learn to listen to its special language, but if you try, your body will speak to you.

┌─ NOTE TO MYSELF ─────────────────────────┐
│ *I will release old pain and seek new joy.* │
└──┘

Once you're committed to caring for your body, you can exercise almost anywhere. (One of my clients suggested that instead of "tightening" muscles, I might talk about "engaging" them.) You can do exercises when you

- walk down the street. Practice tightening your abdominal muscles.
- sit at your office chair. Tighten your abdominal muscles.
- standing at a check-out counter. Tighten your buttocks muscles.
- walk up two flights of stairs. Tighten your stomach.
- avoid airport and shopping mall escalators. Use good posture while walking up and down the stairs.
- visit the grocery store. Instead of standing next to the cereal, stand two feet away and force yourself to reach and/or bend.
- open lower drawers or file cabinets. Bend from the knees.
- stretch. It should have a good feeling and not be a groaning, moaning sensation.

If you get a body signal of pain, exertion, lack of breath, or any other kind of discomfort, something is going on that requires a response. You may be trying to progress too fast. If your muscle gets tired because you're using it, that's natural. It might also be your signal to stop. Or it could be saying, "This is more exercise than I'm used to, so don't overdo it."

People who exercise in my studio hear this admonition frequently, and it applies to you as well: "When you leave the class, take your muscles with you. Use them throughout the day. Don't allow them to remain idle until your next exercise period."

"Don't allow your muscles to remain idle."

When I work with individuals, I observe how they move. Each person needs to tone the body in a different place. If you're currently enrolled in an exercise class, I have a suggestion for you. You own your body. If an exercise does not feel right to you, don't do it. Who knows your body better than you? You have the right to say no to any exercise.

In some situations, you may feel awkward or choose not to do an exercise. The instructor may, in an attempt to encourage you, say, "Come on, do it!" Others in the class may stare at you or ask, "Why aren't you doing the exercise?"

You have the right to say no to any exercise.

Don't give in if you feel strained, uncomfortable, or in pain. You have the freedom to hold back.

———————————— □ ————————————

Exercise your body. Tone it so that you can enjoy life. Toning your body doesn't mean

- trying to match the image of some other body.
- doing exercises with no regard for how you feel.
- being miserable because you don't look like someone else in the class.

Toning your body does include

- learning to get in touch with your body.
- discovering how it feels when you tighten muscles.
- finding the pleasure from relaxing a muscle.

Get your body into the best condition you can, but avoid obsessiveness—which isn't caring for your body. If you exercise to the point that your body is too tired or sore or strained, you are abusing

If you exercise to the point that your body is too tired or sore or strained, you are abusing your body.

You merely have changed the eating compulsion for a fitness compulsion.

your body. You can abuse your body just as much this way as you can by eating lots of unnecessary food. Strive for balance.

If you are a perfectionist or a high achiever, try not to be compulsive about exercise. Otherwise you merely have changed the eating compulsion for a fitness compulsion. You can overdo exercise. If you have any doubts about this, think of the many professional athletes who ended their careers prematurely because they took little care of their bodies. Then one day their bodies rebelled, through sustaining an injury or just being tired out, and said, "No more."

NOTE TO MYSELF

How I treat myself reflects how I feel about myself and determines how I react to the rest of the world.

CHAPTER SUMMARY

Physical fitness is as important as healthy eating habits. Exercise has multiple benefits because it affects metabolism, fat reduction, heart, muscles, posture, and well-being. Exercising should help you to feel and control your muscles. If it hurts, stop; listen to your body. Good flexibility guards against injury. Stomach muscle tone supports Inner Eating signals. Fitness includes posture, shoulders, and back.

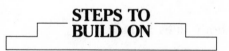

STEPS TO BUILD ON

1. I will seek an exercise program to tone my muscles and remember to be aware of and listen to what my body tells me.

2. I will remember to use my muscles outside class throughout the day.

3. My body speaks only to me. An exercise instructor's role is to give me guidance, not commands.

<u>NOTES</u>

1. Bryant A. Stamford and Porter Shimer, *Fitness Without Exercise* (New York: Warner Books, 1990), pp. 7–8.

2. Philip Friedman and Gail Eisen, *The Pilates Method of Physical and Mental Conditioning* (New York: Warner Books, 1980), p. 15.

Relationships

19

Family Matters

Once the process of Inner Eating began to develop, I saw it would work as well for my children as for my clients. It was a gift to be given in childhood that would keep giving their whole lives. I had read stories and statistics, so I knew that my children could be as vulnerable to media messages and cultural habits as other children.

I was alarmed by the statistics:

1. Nearly one-third of American children (ages 6–11) are obese.
2. Two-thirds of those ages 6–17 can't pass a basic physical fitness test.[1]

However, I didn't want to overreact by laying down rigid rules for them. I wanted, instead, to give them tools to develop internal boundaries, just as I did my clients.

I didn't want to

- eliminate sweets from their eating choices.
- force them to eat certain foods because they're good for them.
- constantly worry that they could become fat.

When Katie was four and Steven two, I questioned the effect of food on the body. I knew it was intended to be fuel, nourishment. But

Inner Eating would work as well for my children as for my clients.

where did hunger fit in? What did it mean to be satisfied? What did various amounts of food feel like in the stomach?

I had to make decisions about the foods I served, the amounts, and my responses when they wanted to eat between meals. For example, when Steven said, "I want to eat," I could have answered him in various ways:

When Steven said, "I want to eat," I could have answered him in various ways.

- "But we'll have lunch in just an hour."
- "If you eat now, you won't want anything at dinner."
- "How can you be hungry? You ate only an hour ago."

Instead I said, "Are you hungry now?"
"Yes," he said.
"What would you like to eat?"
Sometimes he knew exactly, and he'd tell me. Or he'd say, "I'm just hungry, that's all." In that case I might offer a choice of things and let him decide. I consciously avoided labels of good/bad or thin/fat. I would just offer variety.

After Steven made a choice and started to eat, I let him make his own choice. Yet, as Steven and Katie grew, I knew it was my responsibility to teach them about nutrition. I wanted them to connect food with

It was my responsibility to teach them about nutrition.

- caring for the body.
- providing fuel for body growth.
- making their own choices.

Once when Katie said, "I don't like carrots," I didn't try to force her to eat carrots. "Well, let's try squash," I said. "See if you like that taste better." She took a tentative taste, and then I asked, "Do you like this one?"
"A little better," she said and ate more.

I wasn't trying to force Katie to eat squash or any particular food. I wanted her to make a choice based on how it tasted. She could have chosen not to taste the squash, and I would have accepted that. I tried to remain aware of nutritional balance, but I didn't want meals to become a control issue.

I didn't want meals to become a control issue.

Besides teaching them to make choices, I wanted them to appreciate their individual sense of taste. What tasted good to me might not be what they liked. I did want them to have an assortment of foods to choose from.

At that stage, I still hadn't resolved the question of sweets. The more I thought about what to do, the more I realized that my solution had to be consistent with the other things I was teaching them about food. If I could teach my children to like a variety of vegetables and fruit, why not apply the same principle to sweet-tasting things? If I was willing to trust them to make other choices, why should I put restrictions on candy or desserts? My logic made sense, but emotionally I found it a little harder to take the same position with regard to sweets. I did it anyway, though.

When Katie wanted a piece of candy, I let her have it. I didn't make it an issue of control or judgment.

Parents who saw my children eating sweets were surprised. If I was so concerned about nutrition and health, how could I allow that? I must admit I wavered at times, but also I knew that the more we restrict children's choices, the more rebellious they become. I wanted them to learn to balance what tasted good with what they needed for nutrition. Although my style of eating would set the example and play a large part in their understanding, I wanted them to make their choices from the beginning, based on the body's needs and wants.

Dr. Henry Cloud emphasizes the same concept when he writes about abilities and crossed boundaries. I could just as easily have written these words to refer to eating choices by changing the words *talent* and *ability* to *choice:*

> Enormous pain is associated with not being one's true self in relation to loved ones. If loved ones cannot appreciate and value the real talents, the individual is likely to conform to their expectations and deny the real abilities.
>
> The Bible says to "train up a child in the way he should go" (Prov. 22:6), not "train up a child in the way you want him to go." This distinction is crucial in a child's development. We must value the abilities of the true self.[2]

While they were still young, I wanted to give both my children the tools to know for themselves

If I could teach my children to like a variety of vegetables and fruit, why not apply the same principle to sweet-tasting things?

The more we restrict children's choices, the more rebellious they become.

- the feeling of hunger.
- the feeling of fullness.
- the feeling of different levels of hunger.
- the uncomfortable feeling that comes from overeating.

Young children may have no idea how much food will satisfy their hunger.

They learned these four things in a variety of settings. One time when we went to a restaurant, my children talked about feeling starved, so I allowed them to order whatever they wanted. Young children may have no idea how much food will satisfy their hunger. They do know when they are full and no longer feel hungry. Their eyes and their stomachs need to learn how they react together.

As I expected, the first few times my children ordered more food than they really wanted to eat. Using each event as a teaching opportunity, I said, "Think about how you feel right now, after you've eaten just this much. Tell me how it feels."

"Like I've had just enough," Katie said once.

"Like I don't want any more," said Steven.

"Remember the amount of food that it took to satisfy you."

Both of them still had a lot of food on their plates. I said, "The next time you feel really hungry and you think you can eat a lot, remember the amount of food that it took to satisfy you this time. It didn't take as much as you thought." They were beginning to learn the difference between urgent hungry and big hungry.

They didn't understand or learn it all the first time. However, they eventually were able to judge for themselves. Often their eyes were bigger than their stomachs; yet they were gaining an understanding of their body signals. How else would they know what to do when they had too much food in front of them? How else, I reasoned, would they learn to understand the range between real hunger and satisfaction?

One time when my children and I were eating in a restaurant, from across the room I heard a man say to a boy, "Well, you ordered it. Now you eat it. You said you wanted this, so you're going to eat it."

I knew that under other circumstances my children and I could have been in the same battle, but because of my growing awareness of Inner Eating principles, they were learning to make choices.

As my children went through the stages of weight fluctuation, I didn't comment about it.

My children went through stages where they'd be a little heavier, then they'd thin out, get a little heavier, and then thin out again. Fortunately I knew enough about childhood development to expect that. They were going through the natural fluctuations of growing up. When they were heavier, I reminded myself that they were making their choices, and they were doing only what I had been teaching them to do. As they went through the stages of weight fluctuation, I didn't comment about it. Now I know I made the right decision.

"Why would a mother make you eat something if you're not hungry?" Steven asked one day. I was pleased that he had the awareness to ask such a question.

When he was in the fourth grade, Steven bought his lunch in the school cafeteria. He said the person in charge made the children eat the food on their plates. "Why should they make me eat food at school? They don't know how my stomach feels."

"Why should they make me eat food at school? They don't know how my stomach feels."

He had learned to listen to his body's hunger signals, but he still had to learn how to deal with situations where others, thinking they were being helpful, tried to tell him how much his body needed. We were on the right track!

Pizza is one of my son's favorite foods. Because he likes it so much, we talked about how much pizza feels good and how to stop before he's stuffed. Pizza is high in fat but loaded with nutrients.

┌─NOTE TO MYSELF─────────────────┐

Making choices helps me trust my body.

└────────────────────────────────┘

I know that if I had said to my kids, "You can have only nutritious things to eat," it wouldn't have worked. I taught them to make choices about the food they put into their bodies, and that means sometimes they have chosen purely by taste and ignored what they learned about nutrition.

In teaching children about eating, here are a few "Don'ts":

Don't teach them to see food as a reward for being good. (See 19-A.)

Don't teach them to see food as punishment.

Don't label food as fat/thin or good/bad.

Don't make food a tranquilizer and pacifier.

Don't force children to eat.

Don't take away their choices.

Don't make food a tranquilizer and pacifier.

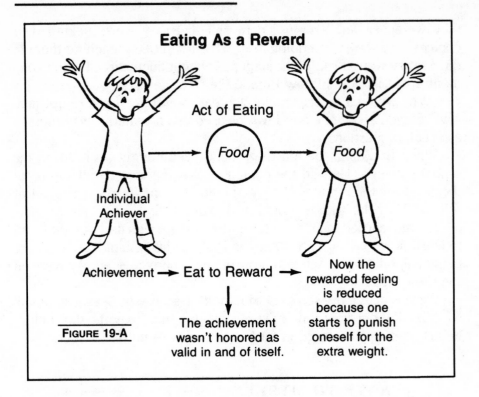

Eating As a Reward

Act of Eating

Individual Achiever

Achievement → Eat to Reward → Now the rewarded feeling is reduced because one starts to punish oneself for the extra weight.

The achievement wasn't honored as valid in and of itself.

FIGURE 19-A

Now that I've laid out the negatives, here are the positive things I hope parents will remember in working with children:

Teach them balance in their food choices, using both taste (preference) and hunger (amount).

Show them how to care for the body. God created our bodies, and we are responsible to care for them.

Guide them in making choices, and help them understand the results of their choices.

When I speak of the results of their choices, I don't mean the old "You'll get fat if you eat . . ." or "You'll never grow up strong and tall if you don't eat . . ." I do mean helping them understand the consequences of choice. They can choose to feel bloated and stuffed; they can choose to remain hungry by not eating.

┌─ **NOTE TO MYSELF** ─────────────────
Healthy boundaries feel healthy.
└──────────────────────────────────────

Isn't one of our major tasks as parents, and those who care for children, to teach them to think and act for themselves? The more we teach them about nutrition and healthy eating, the fewer problems they'll have with food later in their lives.

———————————— □ ————————————

"How do you handle snacking?" is a question I'm asked often. If children choose snacks, what happens one hour later when it's time for the family meal?

The editors of *American Health* magazine and the faculty at the University of California addressed that subject in their book, *The California Nutrition Book:*

Snacks make up a healthy (or possibly unhealthy) portion of adolescent food intake, for "grazing"—chronic snacking both in the home and outside it—is endemic among American teenagers. But there's nothing inherently bad about heavy snacking. It may offend adult notions of appropriate foodstyle—three square meals (with proper representation of the basic four food groups) and no eating between meals—but that is probably not how most of the nation does it these days. Nor are teenagers necessarily grazing on the wrong kinds of foods. Researchers at Kent State University have found snacks to be a significant source of vitamins and minerals (notably vitamins A and C, magnesium, and calcium) and to help raise the content of adolescents' diet to RDA levels.

Even allegedly junk foods have nutrients to contribute. The much-maligned Twinkies are made from fortified flour, which has niacin, riboflavin, and other vitamins as well as iron and copper. These micronutrients and the protein the flour contains make Twinkies somewhat more nutrient-dense (and therefore a better caloric bargain) than apples or pears. But when it comes to nutrient density, there's no beating pizza. Just 4 square inches of pizza contain close to the full range of essential nutrients, most of them at nearly one third of RDA levels.

Parents are right to worry about what are considered junk foods if their youngsters snack primarily on high-calorie candy bars, sodas, and other foods of minimal nutrient density. They should be concerned, as well, if grazing patterns involve substantial intake of fast foods, for the heavy concentrations of fats in fast-food burgers, fried chicken, and french fries can throw adolescent diets off balance.[3]

The more we teach them about nutrition and healthy eating, the fewer problems they'll have with food later in their lives.

"There's nothing inherently bad about heavy snacking. . . . Researchers at Kent State University have found snacks to be a significant source of vitamins and minerals."

"Just 4 square inches of pizza contain close to the full range of essential nutrients, most of them at nearly one third of RDA levels."

Part of growing up and learning to eat properly involves experimenting with taste.

Tastes change. This is especially true with children. Their favorite food this week may be the very thing they turn their noses up at the following week. Part of growing up and learning to eat properly involves experimenting with taste. They also need the freedom to say, "I don't like green beans."

In a family where there's freedom, the table doesn't become a battleground or place for a power struggle over food. The time together then can be devoted to communication and interaction.

When food becomes an issue, children may resist.

For instance, if children can't have sweets, that single food becomes a source of power play. Basically children want to please parents and the significant adults in their lives. But when food becomes an issue, they may resist. In their resistance, they may also feel guilty. Without realizing it, they are often saying, "If I'm naughty by refusing green beans, will they still love me?"

We can teach children by saying things as simple as, "I like the taste of green beans. Taste them for yourself. See if you want to eat them another time."

One mother came to me, and she was quite upset. "My eight-year-old daughter ate between eight and ten candy bars. She was in tears, crying, 'What am I going to do, Mom?'"

"Is she feeling guilty? Or is she feeling sick because she's eaten so many candy bars?" I asked.

"She's feeling that she's done something wrong."

"That sounds like the feeling is in the head, not in the stomach." I went on to explain that she could help her daughter by teaching her to concentrate on how eight or more candy bars felt inside her stomach. "Ask her, 'When did it stop feeling really good? After four candy bars? After six?'"

I made several suggestions that may be of help to other parents as well.

1. I urged her not to say anything to make her daughter feel guilty for her actions: "Use the experience for both of you to learn from."

A few times I've talked with an anxious parent who finds candy wrappers and surmises that the child is eating an enormous amount of sweets. I suggest that the parent pay attention to personal comments about sweets and reactions to them. You may be setting up a guilty attitude in your child toward food.

2. "Figure out why she ate so many candy bars. Do you restrict sweets at your house? Why did she want so many? Help her to think

about her feelings when she was eating. When did she feel she had eaten too many? When did she wish she had stopped? If you put restrictions on her, you're encouraging her to break the rules, to try to get away with something, or to feel guilty."

3. "Talk about the variety of food. Say, 'Carrots have a lot of vitamin A in them. If you ate nothing but carrots for one whole day, that wouldn't be healthy for your body. Neither would eating only potatoes or candy bars.'" The idea is to learn about food—not to feel guilty about it or teach children to feel guilty, either.

The idea is to learn about food—not to feel guilty about it or teach children to feel guilty, either.

4. "Teach her to think and to make the connection between food and her body."

I gave her sample questions to ask:

- "How do you feel as you eat it?"
- "Did you like that feeling?"
- "If it didn't feel good, you probably wouldn't want that feeling again, would you?"

5. "Food doesn't make you fat, but you can get fat from eating too much of any food. Let's talk about the amount of food."

———————————— □ ————————————

As much as anything you do about the food you serve, your attitude is crucial. As a parent, or a parent figure, you are responsible to teach your children about nutrition. One danger is to devalue nutrition in favor of promoting body image. For example, if your children grow up thin, you've done a good job, but if they are overweight, it's your fault. Or perhaps if your children start gaining weight, you concentrate on getting them thin.

One danger is to devalue nutrition in favor of promoting body image.

A daughter's self-image and early relationships with males are often based on her relationship with her father and his views. Consider the effect on a daughter who hears her father say,

"That woman is too fat. I can't imagine why anyone would want her."

"I hope you never get fat. I hope you always keep your figure."

"If you eat that, you might get fat."

"You'd better not eat that. You're already getting a little chunky.

You might end up like your grandmother. You'd better watch how much you eat."

What does the daughter hear? "I want a slender daughter. If you're fat, I won't like you." She may also know that if she's too heavy, he'll consider her size a reflection on him. If he can't accept fat women, he can't accept her as a fat daughter.

She might rebel unconsciously and either overeat or undereat in reaction.

When he says, "You'd better go on a diet," she quite likely hears, "I don't accept your body the way it is. You have to change it."

No one can get away from the fat-thin issue in our society. Overweight children pick it up when their peers tease and torment them. When they put on swimming suits or gym shorts, they feel terrible. Because they don't want to show their oversized bodies, they drop out of activities. They've felt the pain, and they've been rejected just because of their body size.

They may be bright kids who feel okay before the body is rejected. Then, down goes the self-esteem.

As early as third grade, a chubby girl named Barbara got teased and called Baby Elephant. After a while they shortened the name to Baby. Years after growing up, she told one of her former classmates, "No one will ever know the tears I cried. Every time anyone called me Baby, I thought of my size."

After years of struggle with her weight, Barbara has become trimmer than many of her classmates. Now everybody calls her Barbara or Barbie. Few of them seem to remember her former weight, but she can't forget the pain it caused.

This prejudice is evident throughout society. Research has demonstrated that the world is prejudiced against fat people. The reality of fat may be only in their minds; it doesn't actually have to be true. The perception can be the result of just one person's callous remark. For example, a modeling director may say to a hopeful applicant, "You're fine, but you've got to be thinner." The applicant may translate the remark into an observation that she is fat and may launch herself into a compulsive battle against nonexistent obesity.

Therefore, aside from providing the basics for children, we can teach them how to own their bodies. Then if they hear negative messages about their bodies, they'll have strength to make decisions and

Because overweight children don't want to show their oversized bodies, they drop out of activities.

The reality of fat may be only in their minds; it doesn't actually have to be true.

If someone says they ought to be a certain size, they can say, "This is the size that I choose to be. This is right for me."

choices about their body size. If someone says they ought to be a certain size, they can say, "This is the size that I choose to be. This is right for me."

┌─**NOTE TO MYSELF**─────────────────┐

My path might be different from yours, but it's a valid path.

└───────────────────────────────────┘

CHAPTER SUMMARY

Children can use Inner Eating principles to learn nutrition, food amounts and body image. These tools are useful when children eat away from home and when they want sweets. Don't use food to manipulate; do help children to use it in balance to care for the body. Help them understand the results of their choices in a positive light. Snacking isn't necessarily bad. Allow children to learn to make choices. Parents and peers help form children's body images.

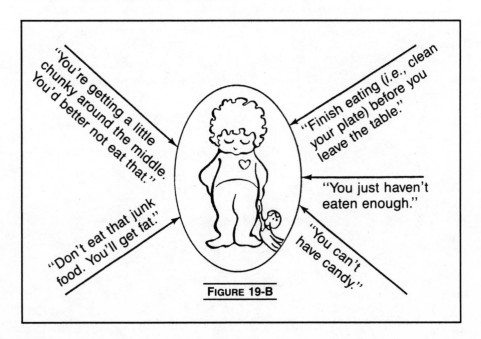

FIGURE 19-B

STEPS TO
BUILD ON

1. Review the basic tenets of Inner Eating, and consider how your guidance can be amended.

2. Consider what body-image weapons were used against you as a child, and weed them out and throw them away. (See 19-B.)

NOTES

1. *Adweek's Marketing Week*, March 13, 1989, p. 22.

2. Henry Cloud, *When Your World Makes No Sense* (Nashville: Oliver-Nelson Books, 1990), p. 153.

3. Paul Saltman, Joel Gurin, and Ira Mothner, *The California Nutrition Book* (Boston: Little, Brown and Company, 1987), pp. 300–301.

20

My Gift

We've been on a journey, you and I, during which you've learned some new concepts, perhaps recalled some painful memories, had some triumphant insights, validated your instincts, and perhaps stopped resisting the idea that you are a unique and valuable person. When I was where you are right now, I felt as if a fog had just lifted. I could see at last.

Before, I had been as muddled as everyone else regarding the relationship between food and the act of eating to weight. Then I saw that my choices and boundaries and knowledge of nutrition fit with the act of eating to determine my weight. It was a smooth system. As a result of that system, I found peace with food and my body image.

My choices and boundaries and knowledge of nutrition fit with the act of eating to determine my weight.

I have been privileged to pass on my system, my Inner Eating process, to others, and I have given it to you. I pray that it gives you freedom and success.

Success in Inner Eating terms means not only weight loss but renewed comfort with your body. When you were a child, you had a good sense of what foods were right for you and how much food was enough. That ability, that sensitivity, is now accessible to you again. It wasn't gone; it was only covered over.

Your right to make choices has been affirmed. Your ability to set healthy boundaries has been strengthened. Each day you feel more self-possessed and more inclined to thank God for your life.

There is no such thing as failure with Inner Eating.

One final word: if you occasionally eat too much or too little, don't worry. You haven't failed. There is no such thing as failure with Inner Eating—only learning occasions.

When you own your behavior and accept responsibility for your choices, you will feel strength from within.

There is no prescribed way for everyone.

There is just your way—the way you choose.

Bibliography

Eating Disorders and Weight Consciousness

Bailey, Covert. *Fit or Fat*. Boston: Houghton Mifflin, 1977.

———. *The Fit or Fat Target Diet*. Boston: Houghton Mifflin, 1984.

——— and Lea Bishop. *The Fit or Fat Woman*. Boston: Houghton Mifflin, 1984.

Bruch, Hilde. *Eating Disorders*. New York: Basic Books, 1973.

———. *The Golden Cage: The Enigma of Anorexia Nervosa*. Cambridge, Mass.: Harvard University Press, 1978.

Chernin, Kim. *The Obsession: Reflections on the Tyranny of Slenderness*. New York: Harper and Row, 1981.

Hirschmann, Jane, and Lela Zaphiropoulos. *Are You Hungry?* New York: Signet, 1985.

Hirschmann, Jane, and Carol Munter. *Overcoming Overeating*. New York: Addison-Wesley, 1988.

Hirschmann, Jane, and Lela Zaphiropoulos. *Solving Your Child's Eating Problems*. New York: Fawcett, 1990.

Hollis, Judi. *Fat Is a Family Affair*. Center City, Minn.: Hazelden Foundation, 1985.

Jordan, Henry, Leonard S. Levitz, and Gordon Kimbrell. *Eating Is Okay*. New York: Signet, 1976.

Kano, Susan. *Making Peace with Food*. New York: Harper and Row, 1989.

L., Elisabeth. *Listen to the Hunger*. Center City, Minn.: Hazelden Foundation, 1980.

Marshall, Edward. *The Marshall Plan for Life Long Weight Control*. Boston: Houghton Mifflin, 1981.

Orbach, Susie. *Fat Is a Feminist Issue: A Self-Help Guide for Compulsive Eaters*. New York: Berkley Publishing Group, 1978.

Polivy, Janet, and C. Peter Herman. *Breaking the Diet Habit*. New York: Basic Books, 1983.

Roth, Geneen. *Breaking Free from Compulsive Eating*. Great Britain: Collins, 1984.

Rowland, Cynthia. *The Monster Within—Overcoming Bulimia*. Grand Rapids, Michigan: Baker, 1987.

Sandbek, Terence J. *The Deadly Diet*. Oakland, Calif.: New Harbinger Publications, 1986.

Siegel, Michele, Judith Brisman, and Margot Weinshel. *Surviving an Eating Disorder*. New York: Harper and Row, 1988.

Valette, Brett. *A Parent's Guide to Eating Disorders*. New York: Walker Publishing, 1988.

Nutrition and Health

Bennett, William, and Joel Gurin. *The Dieter's Dilemma*. New York: Basic Books, 1983.

Brody, Jane. *Jane Brody's Good Food Book: Living the High Carbohydrate Way*. New York: W. W. Norton and Company, 1981.

Saltman, Paul, Joel Gurin, and Ira Mothner. *The California Nutrition Book*. Boston: Little, Brown and Company, 1987.

Satter, Ellyn. *Child of Mine: Feeding With Love and Good Sense*. Palo Alto, Calif.: Bull Publishing, 1979.

———. *How to Get Your Kid to Eat . . . But Not Too Much*. Palo Alto, Calif.: Bull Publishing, 1987.

Physical Fitness and Body Image

Anderson, Bob. *Stretching*. Bolinas, Calif.: Shelter Publications, 1980.

Bach, Lydia. *Awake! Aware! Alive!* New York: Random House, 1983.

Friedman, Philip, and Gail Eisen. *The Pilates Method of Physical and Mental Conditioning*. New York: Warner Books, 1981.

Hutchinson, Marcia G. *Transforming Body Image: Learning to Love the Body You Have*. Trumansburg, N.Y.: Crossing Press, 1985.

Leibowitz, Judith, and Bill Connington. *The Alexander Technique*. New York: Harper and Row, 1990.

Nash, Joyce. *Maximize Your Body Potential*. Palo Alto, Calif.: Bull Publishing, 1986.

Perry, Susan, and Jim Dawson. *The Secrets Our Body Clocks Reveal*. New York: Ballantine, 1988.

Pinckney, Callan. *Callanetics*. New York: William Morrow, 1984.

―――. *Callanetics for Your Back*. New York: William Morrow, 1988.

Stamford, Bryant, and Porter Shimer. *Fitness Without Exercise*. New York: Warner Books, 1990.

Self-Help

Borysenko, Joan. *Minding the Body, Mending the Mind*. New York: Bantam, 1987.

Bradshaw, John. *Homecoming*. New York: Bantam, 1990.

Brenner, Elizabeth. *Winning by Letting Go*. New York: Harcourt, Brace, Jovanovich, 1985.

Buscaglia, Leo. *Personhood*. New York: Ballantine, 1978.

―――. *Living, Loving, and Learning*. New York: Fawcett Columbine, 1982.

Cloud, Henry. *When Your World Makes No Sense*. Nashville: Oliver-Nelson Books, 1990.

Dowling, Colette. *Perfect Women*. New York: Pocket Books, 1988.

James, Jennifer. *Success Is the Quality of Your Journey*. New York: Newmarket, 1983.

Jeffers, Susan. *Feel the Fear and Do It Anyway*. New York: Fawcett Columbine, 1987.

Peck, M. Scott. *The Road Less Traveled*. New York: Simon and Schuster, 1978.

Servan-Schreiber, Jean-Louis. *The Art of Time*. New York: Addison-Wesley, 1988.

Sherman, James. *Rejection*. Golden Valley, Minn.: Pathway Books, 1982.

Smedes, Lewis B. *Choices*. San Francisco: Harper and Row, 1986.

Stoop, David. *Hope for the Perfectionist*. Nashville: Oliver-Nelson Books, 1987.

Waitley, Denis. *Being the Best*. Nashville: Oliver-Nelson Books, 1987.

―――. *Seeds of Greatness*. Old Tappan, N.J.: Revell, 1983.

Shirley J. Billigmeier, M.A., is a fitness and weight-control specialist who has been helping her clients—women, men, teenagers, and children—care for and about their bodies for almost twenty years. In 1980 she founded The Fitness Forum, a program offering healthful-eating consultations and exercise classes to persons of all ages, weights, habits, and histories. She holds a master of arts degree in physical education and health from the University of Minnesota and is a member of the National Body Image Council and the American College of Sports Medicine.